MW01488139

Quick Weight Loss Diet

Slow Cooker Recipes and Tasty Green Smoothies

Kellie Steffen and Jess Brittney Statham

Table of Contents

Introduction

Tips for Quick Weight Loss

Please be aware these are tips for "quick weight loss" but not super fast, like lose mega weight in a week. The truth of the matter is that any diet that claims you can lose the weight uber fast is a lie, or you may lose it fast but you will gain it back just as fast. To lose weight effectively you have to pace it and think in terms of moderation. You must give your body time to acclimate to the new diet and to start the weight loss plan. There are things you can do to help lose the weight faster than with just dieting alone.

Quick Weight Loss Tip Number One

Add exercise with the dieting. Exercising is a great way to help the body to lose the weight and fat faster. Physical activity helps the body to burn calories, which equal to weight. Exercising need not be a boring chore though. You do not have to pay for a pricey gym membership to reap the benefits of exercising. You can do a lot of physical activity right from your home. Put on some good music and dance around the room. Purchase a workout DVD and make a commitment to do it at least three times a week. Take a walk, jog, or run. Hop on a bicycle and go for a ride. Take a swim. Or take exercise classes, you may enjoy the socializing part. Whatever you do, the whole point is to be physically active. Your body needs to be in motion for at least half an hour to make it effective. That is not a lot to commit to, just a half an hour a time at least three days a week.

Exercising is very beneficial in raising your energy level and boosting your metabolism. Because it does this, you will have more energy to continue doing it, which is very helpful in bringing down the weight. You may want to jump in and do it for longer and more often to lose more weight faster. This is just like dieting you do not need to jump in head first with exercising you need to pace yourself. Ideally, it is best to do a good work out every other day for a minimum of half an hour. If you wish to increase this to an hour or to daily or both you can, but it is advisable not to increase it to more than that. Remember, moderation is best, with exercise and with the diet. You will have better success if you pace yourself with it.

When you do exercise, take the time to stretch your muscles properly to prevent muscle soreness and injury.

Even if your exercise is taking a walk around the block, you will greatly benefit by taking a few minutes prior and after the walk to do some gentle stretches with your arms and legs. It is certainly advisable to do these stretches before swimming, bicycling, jogging / running, aerobics, etc.

Quick Weight Loss Tip Number Two

Take the time before you start the diet to wean off the junk food. Chances are you have to go on a diet because of your addiction to junk food. Be assured, food addictions are as strong and real as addiction to pills, cigarettes, or even alcohol. Since a food addiction is strong, it can be tough to stop eating it without properly weaning. If you do not wean from the junk foods, you will experience strong cravings. This is a breaking point for many people who do not take the time to wean. They cave to the strong cravings. They may also have mood swings and headaches that intensify the urge to consume it. Weaning properly helps to prevent these bad addiction breaking side effects.

Take three weeks to wean from a junk food habit. Write down all the times in a day you consume junk food. Then take one instance you consume it and replace it with a healthy snack. Do this for three to five days and repeat the process until you have stopped all the consumption of junk food. If you still find you crave it give yourself a treat once or twice a week as a reward for staying on the diet. If possible though, try to wean completely from the junk food. After a while, your body will crave the healthy food and you will no longer have the ill side effects you did with the junk food.

The best advice with this quick weight loss tip is to think of your diet as a permanent lifestyle change rather than a diet to lose the weight and then go back to your old ways of eating. If you do that, you will gain the weight back. Your body needs nutritious food all the time and therefore you should make the diet a permanent one, a complete lifestyle change for the better.

Quick Weight Loss Tip Number Three

Drink plenty of drinking water every day. Water is vital to your health, while you get some water out of tea, coffee, juice, and milk you need to drink pure clear water as well. Drink plenty before each meal to help you not consume as much food. Consider drinking enough water according to your weight. Take your weight in pounds and divide it by two and that is the number in ounces you need to drink each day. If you weigh two hundred pounds, divided by two is one hundred pounds, converted to ounces is one hundred ounces. A two hundred pound person needs to drink one hundred ounces of water a day, which is twelve and a half cups a day.

Disclaimer for Dieting and Exercise

Always seek the counsel of your health care provider about the best diet plan and exercise routine for you. Go over the plans and make sure they are safe to do with your current state of health.

Section 1: Slow Cooker Cookbook

What Is The Difference Between a Slow Cooker and a Crock Pot?

The old style cookers were called "slow cookers," where the heating element is in a separate unit from the main food holder. Actually, larger slow cookers and "crock pots" still come this way. When the "crock pot" made the scene, it was with the heating element cased within the food holder all in one. If you were lucky you had a removable plug for easy cleaning. Not so lucky were the ones where the plug was a permanent fixture. Crock Pot, by the way, is a registered trademark by the Rival Manufacturing Company, but their name brand became a nickname for slow cookers.

Some slow cookers may have the heating elements that surround the food holder, helping to give it even heat. Others may only have the heating element on the bottom, causing the need for extra stirring to keep from burning and sticking with the food.

Slow cookers come in three sizes, with a 3.5, 4 and 5 quarts being the most popular sizes. Obviously if a recipe serves 12 you will not want to try to cook it in a 3.5 quart sized slow cooker. Most people only have one or two sizes and know how to adjust. Normally, if you have a larger family, you will have a larger slow cooker. It helps to eyeball the food. You want the slow cooker to be filled to at least half way point, but you do not want it bubbling over the top. So consider the size of the foods you are going to cook and gauge whether or not you need a small or large slow cooker. Most of the recipes here do well with a 4 to 5 quart slow cooker.

When purchasing a slow cooker you need to decide first how big of one you need. Obviously if you are cooking for only two or three people, you would do well with a smaller one. If you have a large family, you need a smaller one. Also, consider whether or not you wish to cook extra to freeze and eat later or to have meals for a couple of days. People are finding this an excellent way to save on groceries and energy, to cook a double or triple portion and eat on it for a few days.

When you purchase a new slow cooker be sure to read all the instructions. It will help save you time in the long run and will help to preserve the unit.

Slow Cookers and Food Safety

Some may wonder if when cooking a meal for 8 hours on a low setting, if the food is safe, or will bacteria grow. It is a legitimate concern, but needless for a slow cooker that is in good shape. Most all slow cookers are set for their lowest temperatures to be above 140 degrees Fahrenheit, the temperature that most bacteria are killed. It helps if you are cooking beef, to brown it ahead of time. That way when you put it into the slow cooker it will already be hot. You do not want the slow cooker getting so hot it easily burns the food. If that were the case, you would not want to go to sleep or leave for the day with the slow cooker cooking. If the temperature of the meat is a concern, you can always stick a meat thermometer into it to test it prior to eating.

The Advantages to Cooking with a Slow Cooker

Foods often bloom with flavor if they are allowed to cook slowly, allowing the different flavors to melt together. You know how good some leftovers taste? Well cooking in a slow cooker is like having fresh foods with that have the flavors distributed perfectly.

Because slow cookers are not so hot to burn, you are

less likely to have burned meals. This makes everyone happy.

Even the most inexpensive cuts of meat, which would normally be too tough to eat, will fall off the fork and melt in the mouth after 4 to 8 hours of cooking in a slow cooker.

It saves energy to cook with a slow cooker because, in most cases, you will not have to run an oven for a lengthy time. Running an oven to cook something like a pot roast can take several hours and uses a lot more electricity or gas. The slow cooker runs on a normal outlet and uses less electricity. Some recipes do call for a bit of extra cooking for preparation of the full meal.

One dish meals are easy to cook and easy to clean up. There is no worry with many pots and pans, with having to scrub the stove and oven after a meal. Just clean the slow cooker and you are done.

Tips For Making The Most Of Your Slow Cooker

When shopping for the ingredients in the recipes here and for any foods you plan to put in the slow cooker, consider the size of the slow cooker you have compared to the size of the food you need. If a recipe calls for a roast, try to find one in the shape that will easily fit down in the slow cooker. Many times you can either cut it up to fit, or trim the fat to make more room.

When cooking root vegetables you should lay them in the slow cooker first, under the meat (unless the directions say otherwise). This helps the root vegetables to tenderize better and cook faster.

When cooking a meal it helps to taste test first, to make sure you've added enough seasonings. While it's still bubbly and hot is the best time to add more seasonings if necessarily. Some people even recommend to wait until the last hour or half hour to add the seasonings, so they will burst right when you are ready to eat. The other argument about adding them in the beginning is to help the flavor to disperse throughout the dish. This is where you need to test the theories and determine which way to go. Some meals may be best to wait to season at the end, while others may be best to season at the beginning.

When foods cook, especially slowly, they tend to lose their coloring. You may have noticed this when cooking stews in the slow cooker. You can help make it vibrant again by garnishing with colorful foods at the end, such as tossing in some green scallions, chives, tomatoes, etc. Use your judgment for an added garnishment to add color and a pop of flavor. Not all dishes need this.

When cooking dried beans it is always best to soak them the night before cooking in the slow cooker. If you do not do this, they may be tough and not tenderize right.

Aside from the recipes below, you can cook just about anything in a slow cooker. Dairy-based ingredients tend to burn and stick, so go easy on those. But you can take a cheap cut of meat and put it in the slow cooker and pour broth over it and cook it on low for 8 hours and have a meat dish that is tender and tasty. You can fill it with the ingredients for cheese dip (with often stirring) and allow it to make the dip during a couple of hours. Or fill it with ingredients for hot cocoa and be able to serve a crowd with ease.

You Can Even Make Meatloaf In the Slow Cooker!

You can even cook a meatloaf in the slow cooker. There is not a recipe for this below, so we will share it here. Just make the meatloaf recipe the way you normally do. Take enough aluminum foil out and fold it lengthwise to sit within the slow cooker with enough over the top, to be the handles. You will want to use at least two or three of these, and lay them down so the meatloaf sits on them. Fold them into one-inch wide strips. Mold the meatloaf to fit nicely within the slow cooker. Try to make it where the sides are not touching, but if they do that is okay. Place the meatloaf on the foil strips and cover it. Cook for 8 hours on low, or 4 to 5 on high. You may want to test the temperature in the center with a meat thermometer to make sure it is hot enough. This enables you to cook the meatloaf and not have to be there to watch it like you would in the oven.

Breakfast Recipes

Cranberry Oatmeal

Nothing quite satisfies a tummy like a nice hot bowl of oatmeal first thing in the morning. Often people do not make it because of a time factor. We have taken care of that by putting it into a slow cooker to cook all night and be nice and hot for breakfast.

What You'll Need:

4 cups of water
2 cups of cranberries (dried)
1 cup of oats (steel cut works best)
1/2 cup of cream (half-and-half)
4 teaspoons of brown sugar
4 pats of butter

How to Make It:

Place the 4 cups of water into a slow cooker and stir in the cup of steel cut oats followed by the 2 cups of dried cranberries. Stir in the 1/2 cup of half-and-half cream and the 4 teaspoons of brown sugar. Cook on low over night (8 hours). Stir prior to dividing into 4 bowls. Add a pat of butter and stir. Enjoy.

Makes 4 servings.

Raspberry Coconut Rice Pudding

Sometimes a nice hot bowl of rice pudding just hits the spot in the morning. This pudding is rich and creamy and everyone loves it. It makes a great snack too.

What You'll Need:

3 cups of coconut water
1 1/2 cups of coconut milk
1 1/2 cups of water
1 1/4 cups of rice (short grain brown)
1/2 cup of sugar (granulated)
2 tablespoons of butter
1 tablespoon of vanilla extract
1 teaspoon of lime zest
raspberries (as needed)

How to Make It:

Spray the slow cooker with cooking spray to prevent sticking. Add the 3 cups of coconut water, 1 1/2 cups of coconut milk 1 1/2 cups of water, 1/2 cup of granulated sugar, and the tablespoon of vanilla extract and stir. Add the 1 1/4 cups of short grain brown rice and stir one more time. Turn the slow cooker to high and cover and cook for about 5 and a half hours (or get up and turn on the slow cooker about that much time prior to breakfast). In the morning, turn the slow cooker off and uncover and stir. Let sit for 15 minutes. Pour into a large serving bowl, add the 2 tablespoons of butter and the teaspoon of lime zest, and stir. Serve and top with raspberries as desired.

Makes 10-12 servings.

Turkey Bacon and Egg Casserole

Imagine waking up to the smell of bacon and eggs first thing in the morning and the kitchen will be clean too. This delicious recipe will have the house smelling of favorite breakfast foods. Serve with toast or biscuits.

What You'll Need:

1 pound of turkey bacon
1 dozen eggs
4 cups of hash browns (frozen)
1 1/2 cups of cheddar cheese (sharp - shredded)
1 cup of milk
1/2 cup of onion (chopped)
1/2 cup of bell pepper (green chopped)
1 tablespoon of olive oil
salt and pepper to taste

How to Make It:

First, insure no sticking by spraying the slow cooker with cooking spray.
Prep: Add the tablespoon of olive oil to a skillet and heat to medium. Sauté the 1/2 cups of chopped onions and green bell peppers. Set aside for a few minutes to cool.

Next, layer the ingredients inside the slow cooker. Place 1 1/3 cup of the frozen hash browns into the bottom of the slow cooker. Cut the turkey bacon into bite-sized chunks and layer 1/3 of the package on top of the hash browns along with a third of the sautéed peppers and onions and the shredded sharp cheddar cheese. Do this twice again.

Crack the dozen eggs into a large mixing bowl and add the cup of milk and salt and pepper. Whisk until smooth and pour into the slow cooker over the top of the hash brown, peppers and onions, turkey bacon and cheddar cheese. Cover the slow cooker and cook overnight, for around 8 hours. Alternatively, if you wish to make this for a supper, it can cook in 5 hours on high.

Makes 10-12 servings.

Breakfast Cheese Strata with Vegetables

This breakfast casserole will satisfy and give energy with the savory mix of vegetables, herbs, and spices. Try it for lunch or supper too.

What You'll Need:

1 dozen eggs

1 pound loaf of sourdough bread (no crust, cut into bite-sized cubes)

2 cups of cheddar cheese (extra sharp shredded)

1 1/2 cups of milk

1 cup of tomatoes (plum, cut lengthwise, seeds removed)

1 cup of turkey ham (diced)

1/2 cup of heavy cream

1 tablespoon of butter (+1 teaspoon)

1 tablespoon of parsley (minced flat leaf)

1 1/2 teaspoons of chives (dried)

1 teaspoon of salt (+ dashes divided)

1/4 teaspoon of black pepper

1/8 teaspoon of nutmeg (ground)

1/8 teaspoon of cayenne pepper

How to Make It:

Make ahead 2 days before - First, preheat the oven to 250 degrees Fahrenheit. place the tomatoes, meat side up, on a baking sheet in the oven in a single layer, sprinkle with salt. Bake for 5 1/2 hours. Store in a container in the refrigerator.

The day before - After the tomatoes are ready, spray a slow cooker with cooking spray. Add the eggs to a large bowl and beat, mix in the 1 1/2 cups of milk, 1/2 cup of heavy cream, teaspoon of salt, 1/4 teaspoon of black pepper, 1/8 teaspoon of ground nutmeg, and the 1/8 teaspoon of cayenne pepper. In a separate bowl add the cup of oven baked plum tomatoes, cup of diced turkey ham, tablespoon of minced flat leaf parsley, and the 1 1/2 teaspoons of dried chives and toss to combine.

Sprinkle 1 cup of the sharp cheddar cheese on the bottom of the slow cooker. Next add one-third of the pound of bread cubes, next add half of the tomato mixture. Add another one third of the bread cubes, then the remaining half of the tomato mixture. Finally top with the remaining one-third of the bread cubes and the remaining cup of extra sharp cheddar cheese. Pour the egg batter over the food in the slow cooker, making sure all parts are moist from the eggs. Melt the tablespoon plus teaspoon of butter and drizzle it over the top of the food. Set the entire covered container in the refrigerator for 8 hours or overnight. Next day, cook on high for 4 hours or low for 8 hours.

Makes 8 servings.

Cherry Croissant Pudding

This is a different twist with the famed croissant and with delicious bread pudding. Makes for a tasty breakfast or even a delicious dessert.

What You'll Need:

8 croissants (ripped into thirds)
3 cups of milk
1 cup of light cream
2/3 cup of cherries (dried)
1/3 cup of apple juice
1/3 cup of brown sugar
4 eggs (beaten)
2 teaspoons of vanilla extract
dash of salt

How to Make It:

Add the 2/3 cup of dried cherries to a microwave safe bowl and stir in the 1/3 cup of apple juice. Microwave on high for 60 seconds. Set aside for 15 minutes. In a separate large bowl, combine the 3 cups of milk with the cup of light cream, 1/3 cup of brown sugar, 4 beaten eggs, 2 teaspoons of vanilla extract, and the dash of salt. Spray the slow cooker bottom with cooking spray. Place

1/3 of the ripped croissants in the bottom of the slow cooker. Pour 1/3 of the egg batter over the croissants, place 1/3 of the cherry mixture. Repeat the layers twice again. Pour any remaining liquid from the cherries over the top. Refrigerate for 4 hours. Then cook on low for 8 hours. Garnish with your favorite syrup if desired when serving.

Makes 8 servings.

Hash Brown Casserole

This is always a favorite, the delicious flavor of turkey bacon and turkey sausage combined with the cheese and hash browns makes the mouth water for more.

What You'll Need:

6 slices of turkey bacon
6 cups of hash browns (frozen)
1 1/2 cups of turkey sausage
1/2 cup of onion (chopped)
1/2 cup of bell pepper (red chopped)
1/2 cup of Colby cheese (shredded)
1/2 cup of Monterey Jack cheese (shredded)
1 jar of cheddar cheese pasta sauce (16 oz.)
1 can of mushrooms (sliced and drained 4 oz.)
canola oil

How to Make It:

First, cook the 6 slices of turkey bacon in a little canola oil in the skillet, cool and crumble into pieces. Next cook the turkey sausage, adding more canola oil if needed. Add the 1/2 cup of chopped onions to the sausage while it is cooking. Make sure the sausage is well crumbled.

Spray the bottom of the slow cooker with cooking spray, and place in this order the cooked bacon, cooked sausage and onions, 6 cups of frozen hash browns, 1/2 cups of shredded Colby and Monterey Jack cheeses, can of drained mushrooms, then the 1/2 cup of chopped red bell pepper. With a large spoon, stir and toss the food. Last, pour the jar of cheddar cheese pasta sauce. Cover and cook for 8 hours on low.

Makes 6 servings.

Snack, Dessert, and Appetizer Recipes

Quick Chocolate Nut Clusters

This recipe is "quick" because it only takes 3 hours in the slow cooker. This recipe calls for walnuts, but you can substitute pecans or peanuts if you wish.

What You'll Need:

7 cups of walnuts (chopped)
20 squares of almond bark
4 squares of sweet chocolate squares (baking chocolate)
2 cups of chocolate chips (semisweet)

How to Make It:

Prep: Set out 36 cupcake liners on a tray.

Place the 7 cups of chopped nuts into the bottom of the slow cooker. Place the 4 squares of sweet chocolate over the nuts. Sprinkle the 2 cups of semisweet chocolate chips over the sweet chocolate squares and nuts. Layer the 20 squares of almond bark on top. Place a lid on the slow cooker and turn to low, cooking for 3 hours. After the three hours, stir with a warmed metal spoon or use a wooden or plastic spoon. Evenly spoon the chocolate nut mixture into the 36 cupcake liners. Set aside and allow to cool and harden. Enjoy. (It is okay to set in the refrigerator to cool faster.)

Quick Tapioca Pudding

A delicious favorite, tapioca pudding made "fast" in the slow cooker, taking just 2 hours from prep to finish.

What You'll Need:

2 1/2 cups of milk
2 cups of water (cold)
1/2 cup of tapioca (large pearl)
1/2 cup of cream (heavy)
1/3 cup of sugar (granulated)
1 egg yolk
3 teaspoons of lemon zest
salt

How to Make It:

Prep: Place the 1/2 cup of large pearl tapioca in a bowl and add the 2 cups of cold water. Cover the bowl and set aside for 8 hours or overnight. After the soak, strain out the water and place the pearls into the slow cooker. Turn to high and add the 2 1/2 cups of milk, 1/2 cup of heavy cream and a dash or two of salt. Cover and cook for about 2 hours. Stir often.

Add the egg yolk and the 1/3 cup of granulated sugar to

a bowl and mix with a whisk. Pull out 1 cup of the hot tapioca mixture; allow it to cool for a few minutes. Add a spoonful at a time to the egg batter, slowly to allow the eggs to temper and not cook. Stir well. Gradually add the egg mixture into the slow cooker, stirring to mix. Stir in the 3 teaspoons of lemon zest. Cover and cook for another 15 minutes, stirring every 5 minutes. Pour the pudding into a large serving bowl and cover with plastic wrap to keep a skin from forming. Set aside for at least 60 minutes before placing in the refrigerator. Serve chilled.

Hummus

Hummus goes well with pita chips and makes a great healthy appetizer.

What You'll Need:

1 pound of chickpeas (dried, sorted, rinsed)
7 1/4 cups of water (divided)
1/3 cup of lemon juice
1/3 cup of tahini
1/4 cup of olive oil (extra virgin)
1 1/2 teaspoons of salt
1 teaspoon of garlic (minced)
1/4 teaspoon of baking soda

How to Make It:

First, place the pound of dried, sorted and rinsed chickpeas into a slow cooker, pour the 7 cups of water over the top and stir in the 1/4 teaspoon of baking soda. Cover the peas and cook on low overnight (for 8 1/2 hours) or cook on high for 4 hours. Turn off and cool for a few minutes, then pour into a strainer to drain the water. Pour the drained peas into a food processor or blender along with the 1 1/2 teaspoons of salt and the teaspoon of minced garlic. Turn on and process for just under half a minute. Stop to stir and combine, scraping the sides. Pour in the 1/3 cup of tahini and process for another half a minute. Stop to stir and scrape. Turn back on and slowly add the 1/4 cup of extra virgin olive oil and the 1/3 cup of lemon juice. Put the hummus into a serving bowl and enjoy with chips or crackers.

Chocolate Mocha Bread Pudding

The steamy decadent bowl of chocolate bread pudding will bring your senses alive as you spoon in a mouth full of this delicious dessert.

What You'll Need:

1 pound of French bread (cubed)
8 oz. of chocolate (semisweet grated)
6 eggs (lightly beaten)
3 cups of milk
1 cup of sugar (granulated)
1 cup of brown sugar (light and packed)
1/2 cup of coffee (strong and black)
1/4 cup of cocoa powder
1/4 cup of heavy cream
1 tablespoon of vanilla extract
2 teaspoons of almond extract
1 1/2 teaspoons of cinnamon (ground)
Whipped cream for garnishment

How to Make It:

Spray the bottom of the slow cooker with cooking spray. Layer the cubed French bread on the bottom. In a large bowl add the 3 cups of milk with the 1/2 cup of strong black coffee, and the 1/4 cup of heavy cream and stir with a whisk. In a separate bowl, add the cup of granulate sugar, cup of light brown sugar, with the 1/4 cup of cocoa powder and mix. Gradually add the sugars and cocoa into the milk mixture. In yet another bowl, stir together the 1 tablespoon of vanilla extract and the 2 teaspoons of almond extract and add to the 6 lightly beaten eggs. Stir in the 1 1/2 teaspoons of ground cinnamon. Add the egg mixture to the milk mixture and stir. Stir in the 8 ounces of grated semisweet chocolate. Pour the batter over the cubed bread in the slow cooker. Let it sit for about 20 minutes before turning on the slow cooker. Turn on the cooker on low for 8 hours or high for 4 hours. Check the middle of the pudding by inserting a knife. Pudding is done if the knife comes out clean, if it does not; continue to cook it until it does. Serve in a bowl, top with whipped cream.

Carrot Cake

Here is a delicious carrot cake made from the slow cooker and best topped with whipped topping.

What You'll Need:

1 box of cake mix (spice cake 18.25 oz.)
1 box of pudding mix (butterscotch, instant)
2 cups of carrots (finely shredded)
1 cup of water
1 cup of pineapples (crushed)
1 cup of sour cream
4 eggs (beaten)
whipped topping (garnishment)

How to Make It:

Spray the bottom of the slow cooker with cooking spray. Mix the 1 box of cake mix, 1 box of butterscotch instant pudding mix, 2 cups of carrots (finely shredded), 1 cup of water, 1 cup of pineapples (crushed), 1 cup of sour cream with the 4 eggs using an electric mixer for 2 minutes on medium. Pour into the slow cooker. Place the lid on and cook on low for 5 hours. Serve warm with a dollop of whipped topping.

Makes 10 servings.

Peach Cheesecake

A decadent cheesecake complete with a graham cracker pie crust.

What You'll Need:

1 container of ricotta cheese (15 ounce)
1 graham cracker pie crust (9 inch)
1 can of peaches (chopped 15 oz.)
3/4 cup of sugar (granulated + 1 tablespoon)
1/3 cup of orange juice
3 eggs
2 tablespoons of orange zest
2 teaspoons of cornstarch
1 teaspoon of vanilla extract
pinches of salt

How to Make It:

This is a 2 part cooking, first in slow cooker, 2nd in oven. First, run the container of ricotta cheese through the food processor or blender to make it smooth. Scrape the sides, but add to it the 3/4 cup of granulated sugar and turn to puree for 60 seconds. Scrape the sides, add the 3 eggs, 2 tablespoons of orange zest and the teaspoon of vanilla extract along with the pinch of salt. Puree until combined and silky smooth (like cheesecake). Pour into the graham cracker pie crust. Place an oven safe small bowl in the bottom of the slow cooker. Set the cheesecake on top, if it is not secure, set an oven safe plate on the bowl, then set the cheesecake on it. Cover and cook on high for 90 minutes. Remove cheesecake from slow cooker to cool for half an hour, then refrigerate for another half an hour. Meanwhile place a saucepan on the stove. Pour in the peach juice from the can of peaches along with the tablespoon of granulated sugar, 1/3 cup of orange juice, 2 teaspoons of cornstarch, and a pinch of salt. With the heat on medium, stir and add the peaches from the can. Stir and cook for 5 minutes. Pour over the cheesecake. Serve and enjoy.

Makes 6 to 8 servings.

Soup and Stew Recipes

Chunky Chicken Stew

Nothing is quite as hearty or comforting as a delicious chunky soup made of lean chicken breasts and chocked full of healthy vegetables.

What You'll Need:

2 chicken breasts
1 can of navy beans (15 oz., drained and rinsed)
1 can of tomatoes (undrained stewed - 14.5 oz.)
3 1/2 cups of chicken broth
2 cups of carrots (chopped)
2 cups of cabbage (finely shredded)
1 cup of peas (frozen green)
1/2 cup of onion (diced)
1/2 teaspoon of salt (divided)
1/2 teaspoon of pepper (divided)
1/2 teaspoon of thyme (fresh finely chopped)
1 bay leaf

How to Make It:

Cut the 2 chicken breasts in half and sprinkle the 1/4 teaspoon of salt and 1/8 teaspoon of pepper all over. Place the seasoned chicken breast halves in the bottom of the slow cooker. Turn to low. Add the drained rinsed can of navy beans, can of stewed tomatoes (undrained), 3 1/2 cups of chicken broth, 2 cups of chopped carrots, 2 cups of shredded cabbage, 1 cup of frozen green peas, 1/2 cup of diced onion, 1/4 teaspoon of salt, remainder of the 1/2 teaspoon of pepper, 1/2 teaspoon of fresh finely chopped thyme, and the bay leaf. Cover and cook overnight for about 8 hours. (if you need it faster turn it to high and cook for 4 hours.)

After it has cooked, remove the bay leaf and the chicken breast halves. Discard the bay leaf. Shred the chicken breasts with a fork and replace the chicken to the soup. Salt and pepper to taste when serving.

Italian Turkey Sausage Stew

This hearty stew incorporates lean turkey sausage with beans to make a meal that will satisfy.

What You'll Need:

1 pound of Italian turkey sausage (cut into bite sized chunks)
1 can of tomatoes (14.5 ounce, fire-roasted diced, undrained)
3 cups of chicken broth
2 cups of onions (half inch strips)
1 cup of navy beans (dried, rinsed and sorted)
2/3 cup of carrots (chopped fine)
1/2 cup of Parmesan + more for garnish
1/2 cup of macaroni noodles
7 sprigs of thyme (keep together on stem)
2 tablespoons of parsley (fresh chopped)
2 teaspoons of vinegar (balsamic)
2 teaspoons of garlic (minced)
salt and pepper to taste

How to Make It:

First, add the2 cups of onions to the slow cooker followed by the 2 pounds of bite-sized Italian turkey sausage, cup of dried, rinsed, and sorted navy beans, 2/3 cup of finely chopped carrots, the 7 sprigs of thyme, and the 2 teaspoons of minced garlic. In a separate bowl add the can of fire-roasted diced tomatoes with the 3 cups of chicken broth and stir until mixed. Pour over the sausage and vegetables in the slow cooker. Sprinkle the 1/2 cup of Parmesan over the top. Place a cover over the slow cooker and turn to low for 8 hours (or cook on high for 4 hours). Once cooked, carefully remove the 7 thyme sprigs. Stir in the 1/2 cup of macaroni noodles, replace cover, and cook for another 20 minutes, until the pasta is tender. Transfer the stew to a large serving bowl. Sprinkle salt, pepper, and Parmesan cheese to taste. Delicious served with bread or rolls.

Makes 8 servings.

Chicken Noodle Cream Soup

This pot of soup is hearty and delicious using rotisserie chicken with a can of mushroom soup to make it creamy.

What You'll Need:

1 rotisserie chicken (the kind you buy, already cooked from the grocers deli section)
1 large can of cream of mushroom soup (condensed with roasted garlic)
7 cups of chicken broth
1 cup of onions (diced)
1 cup of celery (diced)
1 cup of carrots (diced)
1/2 cup of egg noodles (uncooked)
1/4 teaspoon of chervil
1/4 teaspoon of chives (dried)
1/4 teaspoon of parsley (dried)
1/4 teaspoon of tarragon
salt and pepper to taste

How to Make It:

First, shred the rotisserie chicken meat discarding the bones and skin. Place in the slow cooker. Add the cups of diced onions, celery, and carrots. Pour the 7 cups of chicken broth into a large bowl and add the large can of cream of mushroom soup. Stir using a whisk to smooth out the chunks. Pour the liquid over the chicken and vegetables and stir in the 1/4 teaspoon of chervil, 1/4 teaspoon of dried chives, 1/4 teaspoon of dried parsley, and the 1/4 teaspoon of tarragon. Salt and pepper while stirring. Cover the slow cooker and cook on high for 8 hours or on low for 4 hours. During the last 20 minutes of cook time add the 1/2 cup of uncooked egg noodles. Salt and pepper to taste and enjoy.

Makes 8 servings.

Turkey Stew

This turkey stew is chocked full of vegetables and fruits to make it a wonderfully filling and delightfully tasty meal.

What You'll Need:

4 turkey thigh (skinless)
2 cans of chickpeas (15.5 oz., drained, rinsed)
1 can of tomatoes (28 oz., chunked and peeled, undrained)

2 red chilies (whole dried)

4 cups of carrots (chunked)

2 cups of cilantro (fresh cut)

1 1/2 cups of onions (wedges)

1 cup of parsley (fresh cut)

1 cup of apricots (dried)

1/2 cup of olive oil (extra virgin)

1/2 cup of raisins (golden)

1/2 cup of butternut squash (chunks)

1 tablespoon of lemon juice

4 teaspoons of salt (divided)

1 teaspoon of allspice (ground)

1/2 teaspoon of garlic (minced)

1/2 teaspoon of cumin (ground)

How to Make It:

Put the 3 teaspoons of salt together with the teaspoon of ground allspice and mix. Take half of the seasoning and rub into the 4 turkey thighs. Place the seasoned turkey thighs in the slow cooker. Mix the remaining seasoning with the 2 cans of drained, rinsed, chickpeas, can of chunked peeled tomatoes, 2 red chilies, 4 cups of chunked carrots, 1 1/2 cups of onion wedges, cup of apricots, and the 1/2 cup of golden raisins and pour over the turkey legs in the slow cooker. Turn to high, cover, and cook for 6 hours or on low for 8 hours. After cooked, pull the turkey meat from the bones and discard the bones. Pour the vegetables into a large serving bowl. Place the turkey meat on top of the vegetables. Add the 2 cups of fresh cut cilantro, cup of fresh parsley, teaspoon of salt, 1/2 teaspoon of minced garlic, and the 1/2 teaspoon of ground cumin into a food processor. Process while drizzling in the 1/2 cup of extra virgin olive oil and the tablespoon of lemon juice. Serve the turkey stew in bowls, drizzle the parsley and cilantro sauce over the top, and enjoy.

Makes 4 servings.

French Onion Soup

A favorite for many, this soup goes great as part of a 4 or 5 course meal or as a delicious lunch.

What You'll Need:

1 loaf of French bread (cut into 8 slices)
3 1/2 cups of beef broth
2 1/2 cups of onions (sliced thin)
1 cup of Swiss cheese (shredded)
2 cans of beef consommé (10 oz. cans)
1 packet of onion soup mix

How to Make It:

Add the 3 1/2 cups of beef broth to the slow cooker along with the 2 1/2 cups of thin sliced onions, 2 cans of beef consommé and the packet of onion soup mix. Cover the slow cooker and cook on low for 8 hours or high for 4. When cooked, pour soup into a serving bowl. Place the 8 slices of French bread onto a baking sheet. Evenly disperse the cup of shredded Swiss cheese on the 8 slices of French bread and place under the broiler until the cheese melts. Ladle the soup into bowls, and place the hot cheesy French bread on top of the soup, or to the side if you prefer.

Split Pea Soup

Split pea soup makes the perfect comfort food on a cold day or a nice light meal on a summer day.

What You'll Need:

1 pound of green split peas
10 cups of chicken broth
1/2 pound of spicy turkey sausage
1 1/2 cups of carrots (diced)
1 cup of onions (diced)
1 cup of celery (diced)
2 bay leaves
1 teaspoon of garlic (minced)
salt and pepper

How to Make It:

Add the 1 pound of green split peas, 10 cups of chicken broth, 1/2 pound of spicy, turkey sausage, 1 1/2 cups of carrots (diced), 1 cup of onions (diced), 1 cup of celery (diced), 2 bay leaves and the 1 teaspoon of garlic (minced) to the slow cooker. Place a lid on and cook on low setting for 8 hours or high for 4 hours. Once cooked, remove the 2 bay leaves and add salt and pepper to taste. Delicious served with corn muffins.

Mexican Tortilla Soup

A satisfying bowl of soup is good for lunch or supper and hearty enough to be eaten alone.

What You'll Need:

1 pound of chicken breasts (boneless and skinless)
7 corn tortillas
1 can of tomatoes (whole and mashed 15 oz.)
1 can of enchilada sauce (10 oz.)
1 package of corn (frozen 10 oz.)
1 can of chili peppers (green 4 oz.)
1/2 cup of onion (chopped)
1 bay leaf
1 tablespoon of cilantro (chopped)
1 teaspoon of garlic (minced)
1 teaspoon of cumin (ground)
1 teaspoon of chili powder (ground)
1 teaspoon of salt
1/4 teaspoon of pepper (black)
canola oil
water
chicken broth

How to Make It:

Put the pound of chicken breasts in the bottom of the slow cooker along with the can of whole mashed tomatoes, can of enchilada sauce, can of green chili peppers, 1/2 cup of chopped onions and the teaspoon of minced garlic. In a bowl, add a cup of water and a cup of chicken broth and combine with the teaspoon of minced garlic, teaspoon of ground cumin, teaspoon of ground chili powder, teaspoon of salt, and the 1/4 teaspoon of black pepper. Pour over the chicken and add more equal amounts of water and chicken broth until completely covered. Stir in the package of frozen corn and the tablespoon of chopped cilantro. Cover with a lid and cook on low for 7 hours or on high for 3 1/2 hours. Remove the chicken and shred with a fork. Replace the chicken, but turn the slow cooker off. Preheat the oven to 400 degrees Fahrenheit. Brush some canola oil onto the tortillas and cut into "chip sized" strips. Bake on a baking sheet for about 12 minutes. Serve with the soup.

Makes 8 servings.

Main Dish and One Dish Meals

Famous Beef Pot Roast

There is nothing quite as special as the smell of a slow cooker of pot roast wafting through the house. Serve this up with a platter of steamed carrots and potatoes.

What You'll Need:

1 chuck roast (at least 3 pounds)
1 can of cream of mushroom soup (condensed 10.75 oz.)
1/2 cup of onions (sliced thin)
1/2 cup of white grape juice
1/4 cup of canola oil
4 beef bouillon cubes (crushed)
3 bay leaves
1 teaspoon of garlic (minced)
2/3 teaspoon of salt
1/3 teaspoon of pepper
1/3 teaspoon of garlic powder

How to Make It:

Rub the 2/3 teaspoon of salt, 1/3 teaspoon of pepper,

and the 1/3 teaspoon of garlic powder onto the raw 3 pound chuck roast. Heat a skillet to medium high. Add the 1/4 cup of canola oil. Brown the seasoned chuck roast. Place the browned seasoned chuck roast into the slow cooker. Add the 1/2 cup of thin sliced onions, 4 crushed beef bouillon cubes, 3 bay leaves, and the teaspoon of minced garlic. Pour the 1/2 cup of white grape juice over the top. Place a lid on the slow cooker and cook on low for eight hours. Remove and discard the 3 bay leaves and chunk up the pot roast prior to serving.

Corned Beef Brisket and Cabbage

This is a favorite Irish dish that can be enjoyed by anyone year round.

What You'll Need:

4 pounds of corned beef brisket (uncooked with seasoning packet)
1/2 head of cabbage (wedged)
4 1/2 cups of water (hot)
3 cups of rutabaga (cut into halves and wedges)
3 cups of potatoes (cut into bite size)
1 1/2 cups of carrots (chunks)
1/2 cup of leeks (cut into 3 inch chunks)
1/3 cup of horseradish (drained)
1/3 cup of sour cream

How to Make It:

Put the corned beef into the slow cooker. Rub the seasoning packet onto the top. Add the 3 cups of rutabaga wedges, 2 cups of chopped potatoes, 1 1/2 cups of chunked carrots. Pour the 4 1/2 cups of hot water over the top. Place the cover on the slow cooker and cook on high for 7 1/2 hours. At the last 30 minutes add the 1/2 head of wedged cabbage. While the cabbage is cooking, pull out a cup of the liquid and place in a sauce pan. Turn the heat to high and bring the liquid to a boil. Stir in the 1/3 cup of drained horseradish and the 1/3 cup of sour cream. Pour into a bowl and set aside. Pull the corned beef out to slice. Place the sliced corned beef on a platter. Arrange the vegetables around the corned beef. Add another 1 1/2 cups of the liquid to the horseradish sauce, stir and then pour the over the beef and vegetables and serve.

Makes 6 servings.

Mexican Chicken Fajita Casserole

The delicious fajita seasoning combined with pinto beans and hot diced tomatoes makes this a meal begging for seconds.

What You'll Need:

8 cups of chicken breasts (deboned, skinless, cut into strips, rinsed and dried)
2 cans of pinto beans (16 oz. cans, undrained)
2 cans of tomatoes and peppers (diced 10 oz. cans)
3 tablespoons of canola oil
1 tablespoon of fajita seasoning
salt and pepper

How to Make It:

Pour the 3 tablespoons of canola oil into a skillet and heat to medium high. Rub some salt and pepper into the chicken strips, then cook for 2 minutes each side to sear. Pour the 2 cans of undrained pinto beans into the slow cooker. Place the seared chicken strips on top of the beans. Pour the 2 cans of diced tomatoes and peppers over the chicken. Sprinkle the tablespoon of fajita seasoning over the top. Cover the slow cooker and turn to low and cook for 4 hours.

Makes 4 servings.

Spicy Beef Pot Roast and Noodles

This is a different twist for the pot roast, with some extra spices and served over a bed of hot buttered noodles. This is an all in one meal.

What You'll Need:

1 beef chuck roast (3 pounds)
1 can of tomatoes (crushed, undrained 14.5 oz.)
1 fennel bulb (sliced thin)
2 cups of chicken broth (divided)
2 cups of carrots (chunked)
1/2 cup of onion (sliced thin)
1/3 cup of tomato tapenade (prepared sun-dried)
1/3 cup of parsley (fresh chopped flat leaf)
1/3 cup of flour (all-purpose)
1/4 cup of the juice from fruit cocktail (canned in syrup, divided)
3 tablespoons of canola oil
1 tablespoon of herbes de Provence
2 1/2 teaspoons of garlic (minced)
2 teaspoons of salt + more to taste
1 teaspoon of orange zest (fine grated)
pepper to taste
6 servings of hot cooked egg noodles (buttered)

How to Make It:

First, add 3 tablespoons of canola oil to a skillet and heat to medium high. Rub salt and pepper into the chuck roast and brown in the oil, searing on each side, about 10 minutes each side. Add the 1/3 cup of all-purpose flour in a bowl and whisk in 1 1/2 cups of chicken broth. Pour the can of crushed tomatoes into the slow cooker. Add 3 tablespoons of the fruit cocktail syrup along with the tablespoon of herbes de Provence and the 2 teaspoons of salt and stir. Add the browned chuck roast to the slow cooker. Pour the remaining 1/2 cup of chicken broth to the skillet and stir until it bubbles, then deglaze by scraping with a wooden spoon the meat bits from the pan. Pour this over the meat once it is all scraped up. Add the 1/2 cup of carrots, 1/2 cup of thin sliced onions, sliced fennel, and the 2 1/2 teaspoons of minced garlic over the meat and around it. Carefully pour the flour liquid over the top. Cover and set on high and cook for 4 hours. Then set on low and cook another 2 hours. Remove the meat and chuck up for serving. Place the meat on a serving platter. Add the remaining tablespoon of fruit cocktail syrup along with the 1/3 cup of tomato tapenade, 1/3 cup of chopped fresh flat leaf parsley, and the teaspoon of fine grated orange zest to the liquid in the slow cooker. Dash with salt and pepper. Spoon the vegetables around the meat, and then pour the liquid over the top of the vegetables and meat. Serve over a bed of hot buttered egg noodles.

Macaroni and Cheese Crock

An old time favorite dish cooked up nice, hot, and gooey in the slow cooker.

What You'll Need:

2 1/2 cups of cheddar cheese (sharp grated)
2 cups of macaroni noodles (uncooked)
1 cup of milk
1/2 cup of sour cream
1 can of cheddar cheese soup (condensed 10.75 oz.)
3 eggs (beaten)
4 tablespoons of butter (chopped)
1/2 teaspoon of salt
1/2 teaspoon of dry mustard
1/2 teaspoon of pepper

How to Make It:

First, add a pot of water to the stove and bring to a boil. Add the 2 cups of uncooked macaroni noodles and cook until tender according to package directions. Drain off the water and keep the noodles in the strainer. Turn the slow cooker to low to heat. Add the 4 tablespoons of butter to the pot and stir in the 2 1/2 cups of cheese until the cheese melts. Add the cheese mixture to the slow cooker. In a separate bowl mix the 3 beaten eggs with the cup of milk, 1/2 cup of sour cream, can of condensed cheddar cheese soup, 1/2 teaspoon of salt, 1/2 teaspoon of pepper, and 1/2 teaspoon of dry mustard. Add to the melted cheese and stir. Add the cooked macaroni and toss until all coated. Place lid on slow cooker and cook on low for 3 hours. Stir every half an hour.

Makes 12 servings.

Black Bean Chili

A delicious comfort food is always a hit. Serve it with corn chips or crackers or even a peanut butter sandwich. This is a perfect recipe to use with a beef pot roast you may have previously cooked, just save 1/2 pound for this chili.

What You'll Need:

1/2 pound of beef chuck roast (cooked and cubed)
1 can of crushed tomatoes (28 oz.)
1 can of black beans (drained 15 oz.)
2 cups of water
1/2 cup of onion (diced)
1/4 cup of Monterey jack cheese (shredded)
1 1/2 tablespoons of chili powder
1 tablespoon of garlic (minced)
1 tablespoon of canola oil
salt and pepper

How to Make It:

In a skillet over medium heat, add the tablespoon of canola oil and heat. Stir in the 1/2 cup of diced onion and tablespoon of minced garlic and sauté. Transfer to the slow cooker and add the 1/2 pound of cooked, cubed chuck roast, can of crushed tomatoes, can of black beans, 2 cups of water, 1 1/2 tablespoons of chili powder and dashes of salt and pepper. Cover and heat on low for 2 to 3 hours. Ladle into bowls and garnish with the shredded Monterey jack cheese.

Makes 4 servings.

Beefy Noodles

Enjoy a hot meal in one with just the addition of a side salad and maybe a roll, you will have a perfect beefy meal.

What You'll Need:

2 pounds of stew meat
1 cup of bell peppers (stemmed, seeded, chopped RED)
1/2 cup of onion (sliced)
1/2 cup of beef broth
1/2 cup of sour cream
1/8 cup of dill (fresh chopped)
1/8 cup of parsley (fresh chopped)
2 tablespoons of paprika
2 tablespoons of tomato paste
2 tablespoons of flour (all-purpose)
1 teaspoon of caraway seeds (crushed)
1 teaspoon of garlic (minced)
1 teaspoon of salt
1/4 teaspoon of pepper
8 servings of cooked egg noodles

How to Make It:

Place the 1/2 cup of sliced onions in the bottom of the

slow cooker. In a large zip loc bag add the 2 pounds of stew meat and the 2 tablespoons of all-purpose flour, teaspoon of salt, and 1/4 teaspoon of pepper. Close the bag and shake, evenly coat each piece of beef. Add the coated beef on top of the onions. Add the 1 cup of red bell peppers and sprinkle with the teaspoon of minced garlic. In a bowl, add the 1/2 cup of beef broth, 2 tablespoons of paprika, 2 tablespoons of tomato paste, and teaspoon of crushed caraway seeds and stir. Pour over the beef. Add the cover to the slow cooker and cook on high for 4 hours or on low for 8 hours. When done, remove the lid and turn off. Let it stand for 10 minutes. Stir in the 1/2 cup of sour cream along with the 1/8 cups of fresh chopped dill and parsley. Salt and pepper to taste. Spoon over a bed of fresh hot egg noodles.

Makes 8 servings.

Shredded Turkey Sandwiches

Whoever loves a good turkey will love this recipe that creates a tender and juicy shredded turkey sandwich with a nice serving of slaw or even delicious over a salad.

What You'll Need:

4 turkey thighs
1/2 cup of onion (chopped)
1/2 cup of ketchup
1/4 cup of brown sugar (light and packed)
2 tablespoons of yellow mustard
1 tablespoon of apple cider vinegar
1 tablespoon of chili powder
1 teaspoon of cumin (ground)
1 teaspoon of salt
1/2 teaspoon of pepper

How to Make It:

Place the 1/2 cup of chopped onion on the bottom of the slow cooker. Remove the skin from the turkey thighs. Mix the tablespoon of chili powder, teaspoon of ground cumin, teaspoon of salt and the 1/2 teaspoon of pepper. Then rub the seasoning on the turkey thighs. Place the thighs on the onions in the slow cooker. Mix the 1/2 cup of ketchup with the 2 tablespoons of yellow mustard and stir in the tablespoon of apple cider vinegar. Pour over the turkey thighs. Place the lid on the slow cooker and cook for 6 hours on low or 3 hours on high. Once done, remove the lid, turn off slow cooker and let sit for 10 minutes. Pull out the turkey thighs and "pull" or "shred" the meat from the bones. Discard the bones. Serve on buns or bread or over a salad.

Makes 6 servings.

Round Steak

A delicious round steak that goes well with steamed vegetables and a salad.

What You'll Need:

1 1/2 pounds of round steak (cut into bite-sized strips)
1 can of tomatoes (diced 14.5 oz.)
1 can of water (using the tomatoes can)
1/2 cup of onions (strips)
1/2 cup of bell peppers (strips)
1 teaspoon of garlic powder
1 teaspoon of garlic (minced)
salt and pepper
flour (all-purpose)
canola oil

How to Make It:

Rub salt, pepper and the teaspoon of garlic powder onto the round stead strips. Roll the strips in some all-purpose flour. Pour some canola oil in a skillet and turn heat to medium high. Cook the round steak until brown on all sides. Add the meat to the slow cooker. In a bowl, mix the can of tomatoes, can of water with the 1/2 cup of onion strips, 1/2 cup of bell pepper strips, and the teaspoon of minced garlic. Pour over the round steak. Place a lid on the slow cooker and cook on low for 90 minutes. Check to make sure the meat stays covered with liquid. Continue to cook until the steak is cooked to your desired done, as well done, medium, or rare.

Makes 4 servings.

Shrimp Creole Casserole

For those who love to partake in the seafood with a New Orleans flare, you will love this shrimp Creole made from the slow cooker.

What You'll Need:

1.5 pounds of shrimp (peeled and deveined)
1 can of tomatoes (14 oz., diced)
1 can of tomato sauce (8 oz.)
1/2 cup of bell peppers (green diced)
1/2 cup of onions (diced)
1/2 cup of celery (diced)
2 tablespoons of olive oil
1 tablespoon of hot sauce
1 tablespoon of Worcestershire sauce
1 teaspoon of sugar (granulated)
1 teaspoon of chili powder
salt and pepper
cooked rice
green onions (for garnishment)

How to Make It:

First, heat the 2 tablespoons of olive oil in a skillet on medium high. Add the 1/2 cups of diced green bell peppers, onions, and celery and sauté. Stir in the teaspoon of chili powder. Transfer to the slow cooker. Add the can of tomatoes, can of tomato sauce, tablespoon of hot sauce, tablespoon of Worcestershire sauce, teaspoon of granulated sugar, and salt and pepper to taste. Cover and cook on high for three hours. Add the 1.5 pounds of shrimp and cook for 3 more minutes. Turn off heat and transfer to a large serving bowl. Serve over cooked rice and garnish with the green onions.

Makes 8 servings.

Jamaica Chicken

Enjoy the flavor of the Caribbean in this delicious one dish meal with chicken and all of the favorite Jamaican flavors.

What You'll Need:

4 pounds of chicken thighs (skinless)
1 can of tomato sauce (15 oz.)
1 can of coconut milk (14 oz.)
1 can of red beans (15 oz., drained)
1 avocado (diced)
2 cups of white rice (instant)
1 cup of water
1 cup of onions (sliced)
1 cup of celery (chopped)
1 cup of carrots (chopped)
1/4 cup of lime juice
1/4 cup of cilantro leaves (fresh chopped)
1/4 cup of scallions (chopped)
1 tablespoon of chipotle chilies (+1 teaspoon, minced in adobo sauce)
1 teaspoon of garlic (minced)
1 teaspoon of thyme (dried)
1/2 teaspoon of lime zest (fine grate)
salt and pepper
lime wedges (garnishment)

How to Make It:

Place the cups of sliced onions, chopped celery, and chopped carrots in the bottom of the slow cooker. Sprinkle salt and pepper on the chicken thighs and place the thighs on top of the vegetables. In a bowl, combine the can of tomato sauce with the 1/4 cup of lime juice, tablespoon and teaspoon of chipotle chilies, with the teaspoon of minced garlic. Stir and pour over the chicken and vegetables. Cover the slow cooker and cook on high for 4 hours or low for 8 hours. Right before serving add the 2 cups of instant white rice, cans of coconut milk, drained red beans, teaspoon of dried thyme, and the 1/2 teaspoon of fine grated lime zest in a sauce pan. Turn to high and just before boiling, turn to low to simmer. Cover and simmer for five minutes. Toss in the 1/4 cup of chopped scallions and season with salt and pepper. Serve the chicken and vegetables over a bed of the rice.

Makes 4 servings.

Jambalaya

Here is a Cajun favorite dish made with both chicken and shrimp.

What You'll Need:

1 pound of chicken breasts (boneless, skinless cut into chunks)
1 pound of shrimp (peeled, deveined)
1/2 pound of hot turkey sausage (diced)
1 can of tomatoes (28 oz. diced)
2 cups of rice (cooked)
1 cup of chicken broth
1/2 cup of onions (chopped)
1/2 cup of bell pepper (green, seeded, chopped)
1/2 cup of celery (chopped)
2 bay leaves
2 teaspoons of oregano (dried)
2 teaspoons of Cajun seasoning
1 teaspoon of hot sauce
1/2 teaspoon of dried thyme

How to Make It:

Add the pound of chunked chicken breasts, 1/2 pound of hot turkey sausage (diced), can of diced tomatoes, cup of chicken broth, 1/2 cup of chopped onion, 1/2 cup of chopped green bell pepper, and the 1/2 cup of chopped celery into the slow cooker. In a small bowl combine the 2 teaspoons of dried oregano, 2 teaspoons of Cajun seasoning, teaspoon of hot sauce, and the 1/2 teaspoon of dried thyme. Add to the chicken and vegetables. Add the 2 bay leaves. Cover and cook on high for 3 hours or low for 6 to 7 hours. At the last five minutes, add the pound of peeled deveined shrimp and cook. Remove the bay leaves. Serve over a bed of rice.

Makes 4 servings.

Spicy Black-Eyed Peas

A delicious main dish which will go perfect with a pan of hot corn bread and a salad. There's enough here to have for leftovers.

What You'll Need:

4 cans of black-eyed peas (drained and rinsed - 14 oz. each)
1 can of tomatoes and chili peppers (14.5 oz., drained)
1 1/2 cups of bell pepper (green chopped)
1 cup of onion (chopped)
1 cup of turkey ham (diced)
1/4 cup of butter
1 tablespoon of seasoned salt
1 teaspoon of garlic (minced)

How to Make It:

Stir together the 4 cans of black-eyed peas, 1 can of tomatoes and chili peppers,)
1 1/2 cups of bell pepper, 1 cup of onion, 1 cup of turkey ham, 1/4 cup of butter, 1 tablespoon of seasoned salt, and 1 teaspoon of garlic in the slow cooker. Place on the lid and cook on low setting for four hours.

Makes 12 servings.

Beef Pepper Steak

A delicious way to serve steak that is fall off the fork tender and tasty.   Delicious over rice.

What You'll Need:

2 pounds of beef sirloin (cut into small strips)
1 can of tomatoes (stewed, undrained)
1 beef bouillon cube
2 cups of bell peppers (red, cut into strips)
1/2 cup of onions (chopped)
1/4 cup of water (hot)
3 tablespoons of soy sauce
3 tablespoons of canola oil
1 tablespoon of cornstarch
1 teaspoon of sugar (granulated)
1 teaspoon of salt
garlic powder
cooked rice for 6 servings

How to Make It:

Sprinkle the garlic powder over the beef sirloin strips. Add the 3 tablespoons of canola oil to a skillet to brown the beef sirloin strips. Add the browned strips to the slow cooker. In a small bowl or cup mix the 1/4 cup of hot water with the beef bouillon cube to dissolve it completely. Stir in the tablespoon of cornstarch. Pour the liquid over the beef strips. Add the can of undrained stewed tomatoes, 2 cups of red bell pepper strips, and the 1/2 cup of chopped onion. In a cup mix the 3 tablespoons of soy sauce with the teaspoon of sugar and salt. Pour over the contents of the slow cooker. Cover and cook on low for 8 hours or high for 4 hours. Serve over a bed of cooked rice.

Makes 6 servings.

Vegetarian Chili

For those of you who are on a meat free diet or who are just trying to avoid extra meat, try this very delicious all vegetable chili.

What You'll Need:

1 can of black bean soup (19 oz. can)
1 can of vegetarian baked beans (16 oz.)
1 can of kidney beans (15 oz., drained and rinsed)
1 can of corn (whole kernel, drained 15 oz.)
1 can of tomatoes (chopped and pureed 14.5 oz.)
1 cup of celery (chopped)
1/2 cup of onions (chopped)
1/2 cup of bell peppers (green, chopped)
1 tablespoon of parsley (dried)
1 tablespoon of oregano (dried)
1 tablespoon of basil (dried)
1 tablespoon of chili powder
1 teaspoon of garlic (minced)

How to Make It:

Add the 1 can of black bean soup, 1 can of vegetarian baked beans, 1 can of kidney beans, 1 can of corn, 1 can of tomatoes, 1 cup of celery, 1/2 cup of onions,

1/2 cup of bell peppers, 1 tablespoon of parsley, 1 tablespoon of oregano, 1 tablespoon of basil, 1 tablespoon of chili powder, and 1 teaspoon of garlic into the slow cooker and stir. Cover and cook on high for 2 hours.

Makes 8 servings.

Chicken and Dumplings

This is an all-time favorite for many. Nothing fills the tummy and warms the heart like a delicious bowl of chicken and dumplings.

What You'll Need:

4 chicken breast halves (boneless, skinless)
2 cans of biscuits (refrigerator, 10 oz. each torn into bite-sized pieces)
1 "family sized" can of cream of chicken soup (condensed)
1/2 cup of onion (diced)
2 tablespoons of butter
chicken broth
salt and pepper

How to Make It:

Add the 4 chicken breast halves, 1/2 cup of onion, and the 2 tablespoons of butter into the slow cooker. In a bowl, whisk together at least a cup of chicken broth with the family sized can of condensed cream of chicken soup. Pour over the chicken. Salt and pepper and stir. Add more chicken broth until all the chicken is completely covered with liquid. Cover with a lid and cook on high for 5 hours and 30 minutes. Remove the chicken and "pull" apart by shredding with a fork. Replace the chicken and add the bite sized raw biscuit pieces and cook for another half an hour. Salt and pepper to taste. Enjoy.

Serving suggestion, add a can of English peas (drained) during the last half hour for added color and flavor.

Makes 8 servings.

French Dip Au Jus

This makes the most tender beef sandwiches and a savory au jus sauce for dipping.

What You'll Need:

4 pounds of rump roast
8 French rolls
1 can of French onion soup (condensed, 10.5 oz.)
1 1/2 cups of beef broth
1 1/2 cups of ginger ale
2 tablespoons of butter

How to Make It:

Remove as much fat from the rump roast before placing in the slow cooker. In a bowl, mix the can of condensed French onion soup with the 1 1/2 cups of beef broth, 1 1/2 cups of ginger ale with a whisk. Pour over the rump roast. Cover and cook on low for 7 hours. Preheat the oven to 350 degrees Fahrenheit, once the meat is cooked, slice the 8 French rolls in half lengthwise (if not already sliced). Spread butter on them and bake in the oven for ten minutes. Remove the roast and slice thin. Place on the rolls as sandwiches. Serve with a bowl of ladled meat liquid or "au jus" for dipping.

Makes 8 servings.

Chicken Stroganoff

This stroganoff is tasty made with chicken breasts and cream cheese. This is a "can't go wrong" recipe.

What You'll Need:

4 chicken breast halves (skinless and boneless)
1 package of cream cheese (8 oz. package)
1 can of cream of chicken soup (10.75 condensed)
1 packet of Italian salad dressing mix (dry)
2 tablespoons of butter
cooked egg noodles for 4 servings

How to Make It:

Place the chicken breast halves in the bottom of the slow cooker. Cut the 2 tablespoons of butter into bits and sprinkle over the chicken. Sprinkle the packet of Italian dressing mix over the butter and chicken. Cover and cook on low for 5 and a half hours. Add the package of cream cheese and the can of condensed cream of chicken soup and cook for 30 more minutes. Serve over cooked egg noodles.

Makes 4 servings.

Spaghetti

This spaghetti is so good you will have people asking you to make it over and over. The recipe makes enough for leftovers or to freeze.

What You'll Need:

1 can of tomatoes (28 oz., crushed)
1 can of tomatoes (28 oz., diced)
1 can of tomato sauce (10 oz.)
1 can of tomato paste (6 oz.)
1/2 pound of turkey kielbasa (chopped)
1/2 pound of ground beef (extra lean)
1/2 pound of ground turkey breast
6 squash (yellow, diced)
5 bay leaves
1 1/2 cups of onions (chopped)
1/2 cup of bell peppers (green minced)
1/4 cup of olive oil (extra virgin)
2 teaspoons of thyme (dried)
1 1/2 teaspoons of garlic (minced)
1 1/2 teaspoons of basil (dried)
1 teaspoon of marjoram (dried)
1 teaspoon of black pepper
1/2 teaspoon of oregano (dried)
Cooked spaghetti noodles (enough to handle up to 12

servings)

How to Make It:

Add the cans of crushed tomatoes, diced tomatoes, tomato sauce and tomato paste to the slow cooker and stir to combine. Add the 1/2 pound of chopped turkey kielbasa. Cover and turn to high. Add the 1/4 cup of extra virgin olive oil to a skillet and heat to medium. Add the 6 diced squash, 1 1/2 cups of chopped onions, 1/2 cup of minced green bell peppers, and the 1 1/2 teaspoons of minced garlic and sauté. Add the sautéed vegetables to the tomato mixture in the slow cooker. Add the 1/2 pounds of extra lean ground beef and the ground turkey breast into the skillet. Turn to medium high and brown the meat. Drain the grease and with a fork crumble it to fine bits. Add into the slow cooker and stir. Sprinkle the 2 teaspoons of dried thyme, 1 1/2 teaspoons of dried basil, 1 teaspoon of dried marjoram, teaspoon of black pepper, and the 1/2 teaspoon of dried oregano into the spaghetti sauce. Add the 5 bay leaves. Cover and cook for 2 hours on high. Remove the cover and cook for an additional hour. Serve over a bed of spaghetti noodles.

Makes 12 servings.

5 Day Meal Plan -

Each meal can be improvised by adding extra bread or rolls, or steamed vegetables, a salad, or whatever you feel is appropriate. For breakfasts you may want to add toast or biscuits and depending on which recipe you may want to add some protein like turkey sausage or a glass of milk. The lunches are soups, stews and macaroni and cheese. These are fine by themselves, but you can add crackers or bread with them. Enjoy!

Day 1 –

Breakfast - Cranberry Oatmeal
Snack - piece of fruit
Lunch - Chicken Noodle Cream Soup
Snack - hummus and pita chips
Supper - Mexican Chicken Fajita Casserole
Dessert - Quick Tapioca Pudding

Day 2 –

Breakfast - Raspberry Coconut Rice Pudding
Snack - trail mix
Lunch - Macaroni and Cheese Crock
Snack - piece of fruit

Supper - Spicy Beef Pot Roast and Noodles

Dessert - Quick Chocolate Nut Clusters

Day 3 –

Breakfast - Turkey Bacon and Egg Casserole

Snack - piece of fruit

Lunch - French Onion Soup

Snack - trail mix

Supper - Spicy Black-eyed Peas

Dessert - Chocolate Mocha Bread Pudding

Day 4 –

Breakfast - Breakfast Cheese Strata with Vegetables

Snack - nuts

Lunch - Split Pea Soup

Snack - piece of fruit

Supper - Round Steak

Dessert - Carrot Cake

Day 5 –

Breakfast - Cherry Croissant Pudding

Snack - piece of fruit

Lunch - Mexican Tortilla Soup

Snack - nuts

Supper - Black Bean Chili
Dessert - Peach Cheesecake

Conclusion

We hope you enjoyed browsing through the slow cooker recipes and hope you have tried a few. Many will become favorites, so be prepared!

It is okay to adapt these recipes and substitute ingredients if you wish. You can add to or take away from, but if you do there is no guarantee it will be as good as the original recipe. But you never know until you try it. You may come up with a new food masterpiece.

Take care of your slow cooker. Clean it well after each use, not just the food container, but the outer body and the cord. Remember you cannot submerse the outer body or the cords in water, so use caution when cleaning. A damp cloth and some elbow grease will go a long ways in making the outside look nice.

Section 2: Green Juice Diet

More than likely, you have heard the term, "green juice diet." However, you may not even be sure what green juice is, much less how to follow this type of diet. Big names, such as Dr. Oz, often refer to green juicing diets. Of course, you may be left wondering what this diet is all about. Why should you even consider this diet and what benefits can a green juice diet offer you? If you decide to go on the diet, how can you ensure that the diet is successful?

This ebook is your perfect guide to making a green juicing diet work for you. First, you will learn what the green juice diet is and how it works. Then, you will get a closer look at all the benefits that green juice has to offer you, and you may even be surprised at some of the great benefits this diet has to offer. You will even find helpful tips that you can use as you begin this diet, helping you make sure that you are successful when you give this diet a try.

Of course, this book is also packed with plenty of green juice recipes to get you started. No matter what flavors you enjoy, you are sure to find some amazing recipes that you will like. Some are sweet and refreshing while other recipes offer you a more savory juice. So many recipes are packed in here that it will take you awhile to try them all out. As you go through and try these recipes, you may even learn enough about green juices that you will want to try coming up with your own combinations, creating your own green juice recipes.

If you think you may have a tough time planning out your meals when you start the green juice, this book offers exactly what you need. After all the great recipes, you will find a helpful meal plan. It offers you a five-day plan that you can follow to get started. Yes, everything you need to make your green juicing diet a success is right here in your green juice diet guide.

Chapter 1: What is the Green Juice Diet?

What is green juice and what is the green juice diet? A green juice is a type of juicer that includes a large amount of greens, along with some other fruits and veggies. The green juice diet is a type of juice cleanse or fast that includes abstaining from solid foods. During this time, you only consume water and green juices. Some people try this diet for a few days while others go on it for a couple weeks. Of course, before trying a diet like this, it is often a good idea to talk to your doctor to ensure it is safe for you.

When you are on the green juice diet, the main focus is providing your body with great nutrition while cleansing out your body of toxins and waste. Greens are very good for your health, but you probably do not get enough of them in your diet. By juicing the greens and other vegetables and fruits, you get a larger concentration of nutrients. It becomes easier for you to get all the fruits and veggies you should have each day. Also, the juice makes it easier for your body to absorb all the great nutrients from the fruits and vegetables.

Of course, to be successful with a green juice diet, you will need to have a way to turn fruits and vegetables into juice. This means you need a high quality juicer. A juicer is the best way to extract all the goodness from the juice ingredients. However, a blender can be used for juicing, although you may need to add a bit of liquid to the ingredients when using a blender. If you currently do not have a juicer, consider spending some time checking out juicer reviews and comparing prices. Then you can choose a juicer that works best for your needs and your budget.

Common Green Juice Diet Myths

More than likely, you have heard of the green juice diet before. Most people have. Unfortunately, many individuals end up with a lot of misinformation about this diet. Here is a look at some of the most common green juice diet myths and a look at the truth. With this information, you will be able to understand this diet better, eliminating all that misinformation from your mind before you get started.

- **Common Myth #1 –** The Green Juices Taste Horrible – Maybe you have tried a "green juice" beverage from a local grocery store and you hated. Now you have the idea that all green juices taste horrible. However, this is not the case. Do not base your opinion of green juices on what you bought at the store. Those beverages have been on shelves for some time and may be pasteurized as well. When you begin making your own green juice, you drink it right away while it is fresh. The fresh juice offers so many delicious flavors.

- Common Myth #2 – Juicers Cost Hundreds of Dollars – Some people have the misguided idea that they have to spend hundreds of dollars to get a juicer. The truth is that many juicers are available for a reasonable price. In fact, it is fairly easy to find a good juicer for less than $100 dollars. A bit of time spend comparing prices can help you find great savings.

- Common Myth #3 – All You Get is Vegetables – This is just a myth. While some of the green juice recipes only have vegetables in them, most of the recipes actually include some kind of fruit as well. Some of the tastiest green juices include both fruits and veggies. Some taste so great that you will be surprised there are any veggies in the juice at all.

- Common Myth #4 – Green Juicing Ingredients are Too Expensive – Before you decide to forgo this diet because you think that green juicing ingredients are too expensive, take stock of how much you are already spending on food. Although produce is not always cheap, it is usually a lot cheaper than purchasing junk food and other processed foods. If you purchase produce that is in season, you will save quite a bit of money. Watch for sales and stock up on items you use for your green juices. Compare the cost of juicing to your previous grocery spending. You will probably find that green juicing does not cost you any more money.

- Common Myth #5 – Green Juices Get Boring Quickly – Last, another common myth about the green juice diet is that green juices will get boring quickly. This is not the case. So many delicious combinations of fruits and veggies that can be experimented with at home. This means that you can come up with juices in many different flavors. Simply look at some of the recipes included in this ebook and you will quickly see that so many options are available for you to try. It will be quite some time before you actually start getting bored with these juices. Once you have tried many different recipes, you can begin trying to make some of your own creations, noting the juices that you enjoy the most so you can enjoy them again in the future.

Chapter 2: Benefits of the Green Juice Diet

Going on the green juice diet can provide many excellent benefits. While this should not be used as a long term diet, using it for a short amount of time can make a huge different in your body. If you are not sure this diet is right for you, here are just a few of the wonderful benefits you can enjoy while you follow this diet plan.

Benefit #1 – Consume a Large Amount of Veggies and Fruits Easily

One benefit of the green juice diet is that it allows you to consume a large amount of vegetables and fruits easily. When you look at all the ingredients going into your juices, you will realize that you could never eat so many fruits and veggies in a single day. If you have a tough time getting all the vegetables and fruits your body needs, this diet offers an easy way for you to consume these foods in large amounts without a problem.

Benefit #2 – Get High Nutrient Concentration Quickly

Another benefit of the green juice diet is that the green juice allows you to get high nutrient concentration quickly. Since green juices are liquids, your body is able to process the juice quickly, consuming those nutrients fast so your body can begin using them right away. Just a few of the nutrients that are found in some of the common green juices include vitamin C, vitamin K, vitamin A, potassium, iron, magnesium, calcium, B complex vitamins and many more.

Benefit #3 – Juices are Easy for the Body to Digest

Juices are also very easy for the body to digest, which is another big benefit. Some of the best vegetables can be tough for your stomach to digest fully. When you enjoy the benefits of those veggies in juice form, you will not have a problem with digestion. In fact, many of the juice recipes are designed to help your digestive system, improving the overall function of the digestive system.

Benefit #4 – Improve Your Immune System

Since green juices include so many great nutrients in them, you also will find that they help to improve your immune system function as well. Most juices include a high amount of antioxidants, which are especially beneficial to the immune system. Many individuals find that going on the green juice diet makes them feel better and keeps them from getting colds and flu bugs as often, since they enjoy a healthier immune system.

Benefit #5 – Helps Cleanse and Detoxify the Body

Going on the green juice diet can also help to cleanse and detoxify the body. In fact, green juices help to cleanse out the body a lot faster than other cleanse diets and fasts. The greens used in the juices help to clean the blood and eliminate waste and toxins within the body. Also, these juices help clean out the digestive system. This means that excess waste is being eliminated from the body. All the antioxidants help to get rid of free radicals and other toxins within the body, cleansing and detoxifying your body as you enjoy the delicious juices.

Benefit #6 – Weight Loss

Many people that go on the green juice diet find that they lose weight while on the diet. Almost everyone at least loses a few pounds, even if they do not want to focus on weight loss with the diet. The body begins eliminating extra waste, which helps provide some waste loss. The body is also kept hydrated and proper hydration with the juices and increased water intake also can aid in weight loss too. While getting plenty of nutrition, you are probably cutting your daily calorie intake from what you normally eat. As you ingest fewer calories, you will probably notice some weight loss as well.

Chapter 3: Helpful Tips for Dieting Success

To ensure you are successful with your green juice diet, it is helpful to have some tips and advice to help you along the way. Jumping into any diet quickly can end in disaster, since you may not be well prepared to follow and stick to your diet of choice. The good news is that here you will find some great tips for success that you can start focusing on before you even begin the diet. The following are some tips for preparation, ideas for great ingredients and more.

Decide on the Length of Time You Will Follow the Diet

Before trying out the green juice diet, you need to spend some time thinking about the length of time you will follow this diet. While green juices are a great addition to any healthy diet, only drinking green juices is not a diet that you should follow for a prolonged period of time. Of course, while some individuals might go on this diet for a week, others may try the diet for a couple weeks at a time.

When trying to figure out how long you will follow the diet, it is a good idea to see your physician. Your physician can give you some helpful advice. The lifestyle you follow may impact how long you can follow this diet. Keep in mind that the first few days may be a bit uncomfortable, since your body will be eliminating excess waste and toxins, not to mention, the diet takes some getting used to. You may not have a lot of energy for the first couple of days, but after a few days, most people do report that their energy levels soar.

It is also a good idea to consider when you will start the diet as well. Most people find that starting on a weekend or during a holiday is helpful. This way you have more time to rest and get used to the diet. Avoid starting this diet when you are really busy or you may find yourself quickly straying from your diet to save time.

Prepare Before Starting the Green Juice Diet

Your diet is sure to be more successful if you take some time to do a bit of preparation before you start it. Preparation is fairly simple, but it is essential. The following are a few preparation tips you should follow as you get ready to start the green juice diet.

- Clean out the kitchen. Eliminate unhealthy snacks and junk foods from your kitchen. This way you are not tempted to eat these foods. It can be tough to follow the diet strictly, especially for the first couple of days. By eliminating unhealthy foods, you will not be tempted to eat them and ruing your diet.

- Get support from friends and family members. Explain to them the diet you are going on for a short period of time. The last thing you want is someone bringing you your favorite foods while you are not supposed to be eating those foods. More than likely, your family members and friends will off you support, and support is helpful when you are following this diet.

- Buy good ingredients ahead of time. Read through some of the green juice recipes before you begin the diet so you can purchase the ingredients you need. Buy enough ingredients to last for a few days so you have all the ingredients you need on hand. If you constantly have to run to the store, you may find it easier to simply cheat on the diet.

- Start eating healthier and lighter meals before you

begin the fast. If you begin eating a lot of fruits and veggies before you start the green juice diet, your body will find it easier to transition to all juices. It is tempting to eat all the bad foods you like the day before you go on the diet. Instead, make it easy on your body and eat light, healthy meals for the best results.

- Work to clear your schedule for the first couple of days you will be on the diet. This way you do not have a lot to do as you begin dieting. Since you may not be sure how the diet is going to affect you, it will be nice to be at home without a lot to do so you can get used to the diet.

Tips to Use While on the Diet

One you are ready to begin the diet, you want to make sure you stick to it. To help improve your chances of success, here is a compilation of helpful tips to follow while you are actually on the green juice diet.

- Tip #1 – Start in the Morning – Do not wait until the end of a day to start your new diet. Begin the diet in the morning, starting out with one of the tasty green juice recipes you will find in this book. This way you start the entire day right.

- Tip #2 – Drink Several Glasses of Juice Each Day –
While you are following the green juice diet, you should
have a minimum of 3-4 glasses of any green juice each
day. If you still are feeling hungry, you can always have
more glasses of juice. Although you want to cut back on
the calories you are taking in, you also should avoid
allowing yourself to feel more hungry or you may be
very tempted to cheat while you are on the green juice
diet.

- Tip #3 – Get Plenty of Water – The juices you make
should not be the only liquid intake you get. It is also
important for you to get plenty of water while you are
on the diet. Water will help keep you from having
hunger cravings and it also is essential for cleaning out
the excess waste and toxins from your body. The juices
are wonderful, but without water, the diet may not be
very successful for you. It is best to get 8-10 glasses of
water each day, along with the green juices you are
drinking.

- Tip #4 – Consider Drinking Some Tea – A bit of plain
herbal tea or green tea is another way to keep hydrated
while you are on the green juice diet. If your stomach is
feeling upset, consider drinking peppermint or
chamomile tea to help keep your stomach calm.
Drinking hot tea before bedtime is also a great way to

decompress and relax, which will help you to sleep better at night.

- Tip #5 – Avoid Adding Too Many Greens – Adding too many greens to your green juice recipes could make you begin detoxifying too fast. Green juices work best when you have 1 part greens to 3 parts fruit or vegetables. You will also find that the juices taste better when you follow this ratio carefully. Sometimes people have the idea that more greens will mean they get better results. However, overdoing a good thing may result in undesired side effects while you are on the green juice diet.

- Tip #6 – Be Aware of Natural Detox Symptoms – When you go on the green juice diet, expect to feel some of the symptoms that come with detoxifying. Some of the common symptoms you may notice include feeling weak, dizziness, headaches and an increase in bowel movements. This is natural, so do not think that the diet is having negative effects. It can be a bit uncomfortable at first to detox your body, so expect a few unpleasant symptoms at first.

Great Ingredients to Use in Your Green Juices

Although you will find many great green juice recipes in this book, it can be fun to experiment with ingredients to create your own little recipes as well. You may find some combinations that you really enjoy. On the other hand, you may find a few ingredients or ingredient combinations that you do not really like. The great thing about experimenting is that you will be able to find the combinations that taste best to you while sticking to your green juice diet. To help you do a bit of experimentation on your own, here are some of the great ingredients that you can add to your juices for great results.

Green Ingredients

- Basil
- Cucumbers
- Kale
- Parsley
- Wheatgrass
- Arugula
- Cabbage
- Mint
- Zucchini
- Spinach
- Limes

- Green onion
- Green apples
- Fennel
- Chard
- Collard greens
- Celery
- Bell peppers
- Romaine lettuce
- Watercress
- Kiwifruit
- Cilantro

Non-Green Fruits and Veggies

- Sweet apples
- Orange
- Pineapple
- Radish
- Tomato
- Carrots
- Pears
- Lemon
- Grapefruit
- Garlic
- Beet
- Jicama

- Ginger
- Blueberries

Other Tasty Add-Ins

- Cayenne pepper
- Spirulina
- Black pepper

Chapter 4: Delicious and Nutritious Green Juice Recipes

As you follow the green juice diet, you will find that many different delicious and nutritious green juice recipes are available. While it may seem boring to constantly drink green juices, the large variety of recipes ensures that you'll be able to mix it up so your taste buds don't get bored. Enjoy different savory recipes or try green juice recipes that include fruits in them, which will give you a sweeter juice that is delicious and enjoyable. While you enjoy these juices, have fun trying to separate the flavors that you taste in the juice. As you drink more of these wonderful juices, you will get a nice taste for green juices. Before you know it, you may be making up some tasty recipes of your own as well. Here are some of the best, tastiest recipes you can follow as you work to stick with the green juice diet.

Recipe #1 - Kale and Cucumber Green Juice Recipe

With kale, cucumber, green apples and more, you will get plenty of great nutrients from this delicious juice recipe. While it calls for green apples, you can add in other apples of choice. Just keep in mind that other apples may have more natural sugar in them than the green apples. The great thing about the apples is that it adds a great taste to the juice, which is why apples are so popular in green juice recipes.

What You'll Need:

4 stalks of celery
1 piece of ginger
6 leaves of kale
½ lemon, peeled
1 cucumber
2 green apples

How to Make It:

Before juicing, wash all of the produce thoroughly. Cut up celery, cucumber and green apples into small enough pieces to fit into your juicer. Add all ingredients to your juicer, juicing until complete. Drink juice immediately. Add a bit of ice if you like the juice cold.

Recipe #2 - Pear Apple Papaya Green Juice

If you like your green juice to taste a bit fruiter, this is a great recipe for you. It includes apples, pears and papaya, giving it a great flavor. You get plenty of greens from the parsley, spinach, cucumber and celery stalks included in the juice. You will barely taste the greens with all the delicious fruit flavors to enjoy.

What You'll Need:

1 large handful of spinach
½ large cucumber
½ pear (any kind)
1 large handful of parsley
1 slice of papaya
2 stalks of celery
1 small piece of ginger
½ of a green apple

How to Make It:

Begin by carefully washing the produce. Chop up the cucumber, pear, papaya, celery and green apple into smaller pieces so they easily fit in the juicer. Place the spinach, cucumber, pear, parsley, papaya, celery, ginger and green apple into the juicer. Juice ingredients. Enjoy right away.

Recipe #3 - Spinach and Kale Green Juice Recipe

Kale and spinach make sure this juice is packed with great vitamins and minerals. The lemon adds a bit of zing while the apples give you a hint of sweet that makes this juice more like a treat instead of a healthy drink. Change it up a bit by changing out the lemon for a lime or two for a subtle difference in flavor.

What You'll Need:

2 apples, Golden delicious
1 cucumber with peel
1 scant handful of parsley
2 kale stalks
1 lemon (or substitute with 1-2 limes, depending on size)
1 large handful of spinach

How to Make It:

Wash the kale stalks, parsley and spinach and allow to drain. Next, peel lemon. Wash cucumber and apples, since you will be leaving the peelings on here. Once ingredients are prepared, add apples, cucumber, parsley, kale, lemon and spinach to the juicer. Process until juice is finished. Drink the juice immediately to get the most from the nutrients.

Recipe #4 - Simple Green and Garlic Juice Recipe

If you want a nice juice recipe that is savory instead of adding sweetness to it with fruit, you will enjoy this recipe. You will get a large amount of greens in the juice and the addition of a bit of garlic will add a savory kick to the juice when you drink it. Of course, you may want to brush your teeth afterwards to avoid garlic breath. However, garlic does offer many benefits, so it is a nutritious addition to the juice recipe.

What You'll Need:

1 large cucumber
1 cup of spinach leaves
2 cups of parsley
3 stalks of celery
2 cups of kale
Small amount of minced garlic

How to Make It:

Wash all the leaves of spinach, parsley and kale. Allow to dry thoroughly in a colander. Wash other ingredients well before juicing as well. Place the cucumber, spinach, parsley, celery, kale and garlic in the juice. Juice. Enjoy the savory juice at room temperature. Avoid saving leftovers.

Recipe #5 - Carrot Cucumber Green Juice Recipe

The addition of carrots to this juice recipe adds some important nutrients, such as beta carotene, that you won't get from many of the ingredients commonly used in green juices. The carrot adds a nice flavor to the juice and the apples give it a hint of sweetness. Avoid peeling the apple and carrots, since the peelings have plenty of great antioxidants in them.

What You'll Need:

3 large carrots, with peels
½ a large cucumber
½ green apple with peel
1 cup of spinach leaves
2 stalks of celery, leaving the leaves on the celery

How to Make It:

Cut the tops off the carrots, but leave the peelings on them. Leave peels on apples and cucumbers as well. Wash the vegetables and fruits well before juicing. Add the carrots, cucumber, apple, spinach leaves and celery to a juicer. Juice the ingredients. Once juice is done, pour into a tall glass. Be sure to drink this juice right away for the best intake of essential nutrients.

Recipe #6 - Energizing Green Juice Recipe

With all these healthy ingredients, you'll get a nice blast of nutritious goodness when you enjoy this juice recipe. It will give you plenty of energy, so consider having this juice for breakfast to give you a great start to your day. Of course, you can always make it at any other time you need a nice energy boost. With the addition of some ginger, you get a spicy taste that stands out among the rest of the included ingredients in this green juice.

What You'll Need:

½ cup of kale
1 inch piece of ginger
2 apples, any kind
¼ bunch of celery stalks, complete with leaves
¼ head of romaine lettuce
½ of lemon, peeled
½ cup of spinach leaves
¼ fennel bulb
½ of a cucumber

How to Make It:

Wash kale, celery, romaine and spinach. Allow the leaves to dry well before you start juicing them. Wash the rest of the fruits and veggies. Add the kale, ginger, apples, celery stalks with leaves, romaine, lemon, spinach leaves, fennel and cucumber to your juice and begin juicing. Pour your juice into a nice glass. Enjoy as soon as juice is finished.

Recipe #7 – Sweet Mint Infused Green Juice Recipe

For those times when you want a sweeter green juice recipe, this recipe is the perfect treat. It's infused with mint, which gives it a nice minty flavor that you are sure to appreciate. The ginger, lemon and mint all complement each other and all the ingredients ensure you are getting some great vitamins and minerals from this recipe as well. With the mint, you get a cooling, minty vibrant taste that makes this juice something extra special when you drink it.

What You'll Need:

1 stalk of celery
1 large carrot, unpeeled
¼ cup of mint leaves
½ lemon
1 cucumber, unpeeled
¼ cup of parsley leaves
½ inch of ginger, fresh
1 medium-sized green apple, unpeeled

How to Make It:

Cut the top off the carrot. Peel the lemon. Core the

apple but leave the peeling on it. Wash the parsley, mint leaves and celery, allowing the leaves to air dry. Wash the carrot, apple and cucumber too. Once the ingredients have been washed and allowed to dry, add the celery, carrot, mint leaves, lemon, cucumber, parsley leaves, ginger and apple to a juicer. Juice the ingredients until completely juiced. Add juice to a glass and enjoy right away.

Recipe #8 – Fill Me Up Green Juice Recipe

As you follow your green juice diet, you may have times when you want to fill yourself up so you are not dealing with frustrating hunger pangs. This juice recipe is packed with healthy goodness that will fill you up and keep those hunger pangs at bay. The addition of a lime to the juice adds a nice little kick to the flavor. The carrots provide great beta carotene while the tomatoes add some lycopene to your healthy juice.

What You'll Need:

1 lime, rind removed
½ celery bunch, with leaves
3 cups of fresh baby spinach leaves
½ carrot top bunch
1 large tomato
2-3 carrots, unpeeled

How to Make It:

Remove the rind from the lime. Wash celery, carrots, carrot tops and the tomato. Wash baby spinach leaves gently, allowing them to drain and dry in a colander. Add the lime, celery bunch, baby spinach leaves, carrot top bunch, tomato and carrots to a juicer, juicing ingredients until completely juiced. Drink the juice immediately to stave off hunger.

Recipe #9 – Romaine Lime Green Juice Recipe

The kale and romaine lettuce makes sure you get plenty of greens in this juice and those greens are just packed with important nutrients your body needs. The apple and lime offer the predominant flavors, giving this juice a delicious taste once it is finished. Try drinking this juice after a good workout. It is refreshing and it will give your body a nice boost.

What You'll Need:

1 green apple, unpeeled
3-4 large carrots, unpeeled
1 lime, rind removed
½ head of Romaine lettuce
½ bunch of carrot top
3-4 large kale leaves

How to Make It:

Start by washing and then coring the apple but leave the peeling on the apple, since it offers a lot of great nutrients. Wash the carrots, leaving them unpeeled as well. Remove the lime rind. In a colander, wash the romaine lettuce leaves, carrot top and kale leaves thoroughly. Allow to drain and dry. Cut carrots and apples into chunks small enough to fit into the juicer. In a juicer, place the apple, carrots, lime, romaine lettuce, carrot top and kale leaves. Begin juicing. Pour juice into a nice glass and enjoy quickly to get the most antioxidants and other nutrients.

Recipe #10 – Vitamin Rich Green Juice Recipe

From carrots, to parsley and alfalfa sprouts, this is a vitamin rich green juice recipe that will pack in the vitamins and minerals you need. The lemon and ginger added to this recipe provide complementary flavors that are enjoyable with the rest of the ingredients. Alfalfa sprouts really add to this juice, since they provide protein, dietary fiber and they have plenty of micronutrients as well, including vitamin K and various B vitamins.

What You'll Need:

2 cups of alfalfa sprouts
½ bunch of parsley
2 carrots, unpeeled
1 lemon, rind removed
3 large cucumbers
1 ½ inch piece of Ginger, fresh

How to Make It:

Wash the alfalfa sprouts and parsley then allow them to drain and dry. Meanwhile, wash carrots and cucumbers, leaving them unpeeled. Remove the rind from the lemon and cut off a ½ inch piece of Ginger. Cut cucumbers and carrots into smaller pieces so they will have no problem fitting in the juicer. In a large juicer, add the alfalfa sprouts, parsley, carrots, lemon, cucumbers and ginger. Juice. Drink right away at room temperature or add a little ice if you prefer to drink the juice while cool. Do not refrigerator.

Recipe #11 – Beet and Cilantro Green Juice Recipe

Even if you do not like beets, you will probably end up liking this delicious juice. The other ingredients, including and apple and cilantro, help to take away from the beet taste for those who are not big fans of beets. All the ingredients pack a powerful punch nutritionally, ensuring that this juice recipe is packed with green goodness you will appreciate on your green juice diet.

What You'll Need:

5 leaves of romaine lettuce, large
½ bunch of Cilantro
½ green apple (like Granny Smith)
1 lime, rind removed
1 beet
3-4 kale leaves, large
2 cups of fresh spinach leaves

How to Make It:

Wash the romaine lettuce, cilantro, kale leaves and spinach leaves. Use a colander and then allow greens to drain and dry. Meanwhile, core the green apple. Remove the rind from the lime and then wash and prepare the beet for juicing. Cut up any pieces that are too large for your juicer to ensure everything fits without a problem. Add all ingredients, the romaine lettuce, cilantro, green apple, lime, beet, kale leaves and spinach leaves, to a juicer. Juice the ingredients. Add to a large glass and then enjoy drinking the delicious juice right away.

Recipe #12 – Broccoli Wheatgrass Green Juice Recipe

Wheatgrass has so many great benefits. For example, it is known to help detoxify the body. It also offers great enzymes and works to neutralize toxins in the body. Wheatgrass also includes many important minerals and vitamins, including calcium, iron, beta carotene and important amino acids that the body needs. Broccoli also has plenty of vitamins and minerals, not to mention the natural goodness you'll get from the cucumber, cabbage and apple included in this recipe.

What You'll Need:

1 beet
1 green apple, unpeeled
1 cucumber
1 large handful of spinach leaves
1 inch of wheatgrass
1 stalk of broccoli
1 cup of cabbage

How to Make It:

Wash the wheatgrass carefully and place on a paper towel to dry. Wash spinach and cabbage in a colander, allowing it to drain and finish drying before juicing. Wash and core the apple but leave the peeling on it. The beet, broccoli and cucumber should all be washed as well. Cut the broccoli, beet, cucumber and apple into chunks. Place the beet, green apple, cucumber, spinach leaves, wheatgrass, broccoli and cabbage into a juicer. Begin juicing. Once finished, pour juice into a tall glass. Kick back and enjoy this delicious, nutritious juice.

Recipe #13 – Easy Cucumber Salad Green Juice Recipe

If you are a big fan of all the flavors in a delicious cucumber salad, you are sure to love this green juice recipe. It has all the flavors that you would expect in cucumber salad, giving it a nice, full bodied flavor. While the recipe doesn't call for basil, you could always add a couple leaves of basil to the recipe, enhancing the flavor of the cucumbers, romaine and tomatoes even more.

What You'll Need:

3 large leaves of romaine lettuce
2-3 tomatoes, medium sized
½ small lemon, rind removed
1 large cucumber, unpeeled

How to Make It:

Start by washing the romaine leaves very gently and allowing them to dry. Meanwhile, remove the rind from the ½ lemon. Wash the tomatoes and the cucumber, leaving the peel on the cucumber. Cut up the cucumber and tomatoes into large chunks so they will easily go through your juicer without a problem.

Recipe #14 – Celery Cucumber Spinach Green Juice Recipe

This juice has a very green, healthy flavor to it and all the spinach adds plenty of nutrients. If you try the juice and you are not happy with the flavor, try adding a bit of lemon to the juice, which will give it a nice tang. Simply adding half of a lemon should be plenty of you want that tangy flavor.

What You'll Need:

2 celery stalks with the leaves in tact
1 cucumber, unpeeled
2 large handfuls of baby spinach (or regular spinach if you do not have baby spinach on hand)

How to Make It:

Wash the spinach leaves carefully, draining them well before juicing. Wash the celery stalks and the cucumber well. Cut the celery stalks and cucumber into large chunks. Begin by adding the spinach to the juicer, juicing it alone first. Next, add the cucumber and celery stalks to the juicer and juice. The cucumber will help clean out the rest of the spinach left in the juicer, making sure you make the most of the nutrients found in the spinach.

Serve in a glass and drink immediately.

Recipe #15 – Zucchini Cucumber Green Juice Recipe

If you need a great afternoon snack, you may want to try this green juice recipe. It is packed with hearty veggies that will keep you feeling full while providing a nice boost of nutrition. It should give you some extra energy if you often feel tired in the late afternoon as well.

What You'll Need:

1 large handful of spinach
1 cucumber, unpeeled
1 beet
1 zucchini, unpeeled
4 celery stalks

How to Make It:

Wash spinach in a large colander, allowing it to drain and dry. Wash the celery, beet, cucumber and zucchini well. For best results, wash produce for about 30 seconds. Chop up the cucumber, beet, zucchini and celery into large chunks to fit the size of your juicer. Place the veggies, spinach, cucumber, beet, zucchini and celery, into the juicer. Juice veggies. Serve in a nice glass and enjoy the green juice snack.

Recipe #16 – Cabbage Broccoli Green Juice Recipe for Better Digestion

The right combination of veggies can help improve your digestion, meaning that your green juice will give you plenty of great vitamins and minerals while ensuring that your digestive system is working at its best. The combination of these ingredients, including broccoli and cabbage, makes a nice juice with plenty of great flavor. If you need a little extra flavor, you can add a little spritz of lemon juice, cayenne pepper or even a bit of licorice root to the recipe.

What You'll Need:

1 large stalk of broccoli
3 large carrots, unpeeled
¼ head of green cabbage
1 medium sized tomato

How to Make It:

Wash all of the vegetables. Leave peel on the carrots. Chop all veggies into large pieces, ensuring the pieces will fit nicely in your juicer. Add the broccoli, unpeeled carrots, green cabbage and tomato (also unpeeled and unseeded) to the juicer. Juice the ingredients. Enjoy whenever you feel your digestive system needs a bit of a boost.

Recipe #17 – Watermelon and Cabbage Green Juice Recipe with Honey

The cabbage adds plenty of greens to this juice, but you also get some wonderful fruits in the juice with the addition of an apple and some watermelon. The recipe calls for a bit of honey, which is not added to the juice until after all the produce has been juiced. If you do not want to use honey in your juice, simply leave it out. It will not cause a problem with the recipe.

What You'll Need:

1 green apple, unpeeled
2 large carrots, unpeeled
1/3 head of white cabbage
1 teaspoon of honey
2 cups of watermelon, cubed

How to Make It:

Take the cabbage and separate the leaves. Once leaves are separated, clean them thoroughly. Wash the carrots and the apple, leaving the peelings on. Remove the core from the apple and remove the tops from the carrots. Cut carrots and apple into large cubes. Add the apple, carrots, white cabbage and watermelon to the juicer.

Juice the ingredients. Add juice to a large glass. Stir in the honey and then enjoy immediately.

Recipe #18 – Easy Apple Wheatgrass Green Juice Recipe

This recipe is one of the easiest green juice recipes to make. Wheatgrass is so good for you, providing you with many important vitamins and minerals that are needed in your body. However, many people do not like the taste of wheatgrass. Adding the apple to the wheatgrass will help to mask the flavor of wheatgrass, making a tasty juice that you will enjoy. Before juicing wheatgrass, make sure your juicer will juice wheatgrass without a problem.

What You'll Need:

2 large Granny Smith green apples
2 inches of wheatgrass

How to Make It:

Wash the wheat grass carefully and allow to dry. Wash the apples and then remove their cores. However, make sure you do leave the peels on the apples for more nutrients in the juice. Place the wheatgrass and the apples into the juicer, chunking apples if they are too large. Juice. Drink right away for the best benefits.

Recipe #19 – Spinach and Orange Green Juice Recipe

Spinach is one of the best ingredients to use in green juices, but some individuals feel that the flavor it provides is a bit too green. With this recipe, you get a lot of spinach and all the goodness it has to offer. However, an orange is also used in this green juice, which gives it a nice citrus flavor, along with the carrots also used in the recipe. This delicious juice is perfect early in the morning. Skip the orange juice and go with this spinach and orange green juice recipe – it is much better for you.

What You'll Need:

2-3 large carrots, unpeeled
3-4 large handfuls of spinach leaves
1 cucumber, unpeeled
1 large orange, rind removed

How to Make It:

Store all ingredients in the refrigerator before preparing them for juicing. Wash the spinach gently in cool water and allow to drain a bit in a colander before juicing it. Peel the orange, leaving a bit of the white behind. Wash the carrots and the cucumber well, but leave them both unpeeled. Break the orange into sections and chop the carrots and cucumber into chunks. Put the carrots, spinach leaves, cucumber and the orange into the juicer, juicing until completed. Serve right away while cool. If the juice isn't cool enough, add a bit of ice to the glass for a nice, chilling, refreshing drink.

Recipe #20 – Antioxidant Citrus and Spinach Green Juice Recipe

Citrus fruits have plenty of antioxidants, especially vitamin C. Spinach is also very high in minerals, phytonutrients and vitamins. Some of the great vitamins included in spinach include vitamin C, vitamin K, vitamin B6, vitamin A and vitamin B2. It also provides other important nutrients your body needs, such as copper, phosphorus, iron, magnesium, calcium and manganese. All the spinach in this recipe combined with citrus fruits provides a powerful antioxidant punch. This is a great recipe to use if you feel like you may be catching a cold or getting the flu, since it will give your immune system a good boost.

What You'll Need:

2 stalks of celery with the leaves
1 large grapefruit, rind removed
¼ beet
2 large handfuls of spinach leaves
1 medium sized carrot, unpeeled
1 large orange, rind removed

How to Make It:

Get started with the preparation by washing the spinach to remove any dirt or pesticides (using organic is best and eliminates the risk of pesticides on your produce). Make sure spinach has a bit of time to dry. Peel the grapefruit and the orange, dividing into sections. Prepare the beet, making sure you only use a quarter of the beet for the recipe. Wash celery and carrot, leaving the peel on the carrot. Chop carrot and celery into large chunks. Add celery, grapefruit, beet, spinach leaves, carrot and orange into the juicer. Juice ingredients. Fill a large glass with ice, pouring juice over ice for a delicious citrus juice that is nice and cold.

Recipe #21 – Tropical Sweet Kale Green Juice Recipe

This recipe includes a large amount of kale, which is very low on calories, while providing plenty of fiber, vitamins and minerals. Kale also is high in antioxidants, such as Vitamin A and Vitamin C. Surprisingly to many, omega-3 fatty acids are also found in kale, helping to fight off inflammation in the body. In fact, some studies show that kale's anti-inflammatory and antioxidant qualities may help to combat and prevent certain types of cancer, including ovarian, breast, prostate, colon and bladder cancers. The addition of tropical fruits, green apple and a pear give this juice a surprising sweet taste that you are sure to enjoy.

What You'll Need:

1 large cucumber, unpeeled
3 large spinach leaves
6-10 large kale leaves
1 green pear
1 cup of papaya, chopped
1 large orange, with rind removed
1 large green apple, unpeeled

How to Make It:

In a colander, rinse off the spinach and kale leaves. Leave in colander to drain. Meanwhile, peel the orange and pull apart into several large pieces. Wash the cucumber, pear and green apple. Core the green apple. Remove seed and core area from the pear. Cut cucumber, pear and green apple into large chunks.

Combine together the cucumber, spinach leaves, kale leaves, pear, papaya, orange and green apple in the juicer. Begin juicing. When juice is complete, serve this juice over ice for a sweet green juice that is cold and refreshing. Some people prefer to thin the juice just a bit with a little bit of filtered water. If you have leftovers, store covered in the refrigerator and drink within 8 hours or less.

Recipe #22 – Carrot and Kale Green Juice Recipe

Here you have another great green juice recipe that uses kale. Kales offers many vitamins, such as Vitamin K, A and C. Carrots add beta carotene to the juice, as well as many other important nutrients. The bits of orange and lemon juice add a little bit of citrus zing to the juice. The apple, orange and lemon all help to mellow the kale flavor out a bit, making a tastier juice.

What You'll Need:

3 medium sized carrots, unpeeled
¼ beet
3 large leaves of kale
½ orange, rind removed
2 celery stalks with leaves
½ medium sized green apple
½ lemon, rind removed

How to Make It:

Gently place kale leaves in a colander, rinsing them carefully to clean them. While kale is drying, prepare ¼ beet, covering the rest of the beet to use in another juice recipe later. Peel the rind off the lemon and the orange. Separate the orange into sections. Wash the carrots, celery and green apple. Leave the carrots unpeeled but cut off the tops. Cut the carrots up into chunks. Core the apple, chunk up half of the apple, saving the rest for another recipe or a snack later.

Next, carrots, ¼ beet, kale leaves, orange, celery, green apple and lemon should all be added to your juicer. Juice the ingredients until the juicing is complete. Fill a glass halfway with crushed ice. Pour the carrot and kale green juice over the crushed ice, drinking it right away.

Recipe #23 – Italian Style Green Juice Recipe

This tasty recipe uses a lot of veggies that are used in Italian dishes. The combination goes together well and the basil leaves really adds big flavor to this wonderful juice. Keep in mind, the basil and parsley used in the recipe are not to be juiced. Instead, they are added into the juice at the end, right before you begin drinking it. With this Italian style green juice, you can help fix that craving for Italian food the healthy way.

What You'll Need:

2 large bell peppers of any color
2 large tomatoes
3 large carrots, unpeeled
1 large handful of spinach leaves
4 leaves of fresh basil
1 celery stalk with leaves on it
1 large handful of fresh flat leaf parsley

How to Make It:

Begin by placing the handful of spinach leaves into a colander so they can easily be washed and allowed to dry a bit. After washing spinach, wash the peppers, tomatoes, carrots and celery. Once spinach is dry, remove it and add basil and flat leaf parsley to the colander, washing it carefully. Cut up bell peppers, removing seeds and insides. Cut peppers into large chunks. Cut tomatoes into chunks, leaving skin and seeds in place. Cut the tops off the carrots, leave the peels on and then chop carrots into large pieces. Celery should also be chopped into big pieces that will fit in the juicer you have on hand.

Place the bell peppers, tomatoes, carrots, spinach leaves and celery in the juicer. Juice veggies. Pour juice into a tall glass. Chop up the basil and flat leaf parsley roughly. Add basil and parsley to the juice, stirring it in well. Drink right away and enjoy.

Recipe #24 – Bell Pepper Beet and Kale Green Juice Recipe

You probably already know how great kale is for you, with all the great vitamins it includes, not to mention the high amount of fiber and included omega 3s. However, you may not realize how good beets are for you. They naturally contain beta carotene, a lot of fiber, iron, vitamin A, vitamin C, folic acid, certain B vitamins, potassium and magnesium. They are excellent for cleansing the body, cleaning the blood and helping out the liver as well. Of course, the tomatoes and bell pepper add even more great nutrients.

What You'll Need:

½ bell pepper of any color
1 beet
½ medium sized lemon, rind removed
1 large bunch of kale
4 large tomatoes
¼ cup of purified water

How to Make It:

Wash all the kale carefully. Using a colander helps and you can leave it in the colander to drain and dry a bit while you work with the other ingredients. Peel the beet, chopping off the tail and the top. Cut up the beet into chunks. Wash the bell pepper, removing seeds and cutting up half the pepper into chunks. Cut a lemon in half, removing the find from the half you plan to use in the juice. Wash tomatoes, chopping them into large pieces as well.

The bell pepper, beet, lemon, kale and tomatoes should all be placed into your juicer. Juice the ingredients until the juicer has finished. Pour the juice into a glass large enough to fit in a bit more liquid. Add the purified water. Mix into the juice well. Drink and enjoy.

Recipe #25 – Delicious Watercress Green Bean and Spinach Green Juice Recipe

Green beans help to cleanse out the body and also help with weight loss. The watercress in the recipe is known to help neutralize toxins, clean out intestines and help to stimulate fat burning within the body. Spinach has a lot of chlorophyll in it, which works to cleanse the body as well, also helping to help with lymph and blood circulation. The other ingredients in this green juice recipe, such as apples an cucumbers, also have many benefits that really make this recipe a powerful one you will want to try.

What You'll Need:

2 large handfuls of baby spinach leaves
1 small bunch of watercress
1 handful of green beans, fresh
1 large Granny Smith green apple, unpeeled
1 large cucumber
1 large carrot, unpeeled
½ lemon, rind removed

How to Make It:

In a colander, begin by washing the watercress and the

baby spinach leaves. Leave both in the colander to drain the excess water away. Wash green beans, then remove the ends and break them in half. Wash the Granny Smith apple. Core the apple, and then cut into chunks. Do not remove the apple's skin. Wash the cucumber and carrots. Remove the top from the carrot. Leave both the cucumber and carrot unpeeled, cutting them up into big pieces. Peel the lemon, cutting it in half. Store the other half in the refrigerator to use later.

In a large juicer, place the baby spinach leaves, watercress and the green beans. Juice. Next, add the apple, cucumber, carrot and lemon to the juicer. Juice these ingredients. The second juicing will clean out what is left of the spinach and watercress leaves, ensuring you get all the nutrients these leaves have to offer you. Serve the juice right away, enjoying the natural goodness.

Recipe #26 – Tangerine Broccoli Green Juice with Ginger Recipe

Broccoli packs a powerful nutritious punch, making it a great base for this green juice recipe. The addition of the tangerines adds even more great nutrients. Tangerines have a lot of vitamin C in them and the pectin in this fruit helps to improve digestion as well. You'll also find that tangerines have calcium and vitamin C in them, while they are low in fat and calories. By adding the tangerines, you not only add more nutrients, but you also add some great flavor to this juice, which will tempt your taste buds.

What You'll Need:

2 large tangerines, seeds and rind removed
½ teaspoon of grated ginger, fresh
4 stalks of celery, leave the leaves on
8 florets of broccoli
2-4 ounces of filtered water

How to Make It:

Peel the tangerines and then pull them into sections, removing any seeds you find. Wash the celery stalks and then chop. Wash the broccoli florists carefully, chopping the broccoli into pieces as well. Add the tangerine sections, celery pieces and chunks of broccoli to the juicer. Juice ingredients. Once juice is complete, pour juice into a big glass. Add the filtered water to taste, mixing well. Mix in the grated ginger and then consume the juice right away.

Recipe #27 – Strawberry and Tangerine Green Juice Recipe

Both the kale and the spinach included in this recipe include plenty of excellent vitamins and minerals. The tangerines add vitamin C. The strawberries included in this green juice really help add more vitamins and other nutrients to the juice. Not only are strawberries high in vitamin C, but they also happen to be a great source of vitamin B6, vitamin K, magnesium, folic acid, riboflavin, copper, omega 3s, vitamin B5 and potassium. Strawberries are good for you, but they also taste great and make this green juice recipe something special.

What You'll Need:

2 cups of fresh baby spinach
10 leaves of kale
1 large tangerine, rind and seeds removed
2-4 ounces of filtered water
1 cup of whole strawberries

How to Make It:

Fill a colander with the baby spinach and kale, rinsing for a couple minutes with cold water. Leave in the colander to dry. Meanwhile, peel the tangerine. Break apart the sections of the tangerines, pulling out any seeds. You definitely do not want tangerine seeds in your juicer. Wash the strawberries thoroughly. Then, cut the tops off the strawberries, but leave them whole. Add the baby spinach, kale, tangerine and the strawberries to a juicer. Begin juicing. Once the juice is ready, pour into a big cup. Mix in the filtered water until well combined. Drink the juice. If you prefer it cold, add a bit of ice to the glass for a cool, fruity green juice.

Recipe #28 – Pineapple Orange Green Juice Recipe

When you drink this green juice, you'll barely know that there is any spinach in it because of the wonderful flavors provided by the pineapple and orange combination. With the addition of the pineapple, you get many nutritional benefits. First, pineapple offers more than 100% of a daily serving of vitamin C, which is an important antioxidant. It also contains bromelain, which is an enzyme that helps to relive inflammation in the body. Plenty of fiber is found in this fruit as well, which helps the colon and digestive system. This is a recipe that tastes amazing cold, so refrigerate ingredients before juicing and consider adding a bit of ice to make it extra cold.

What You'll Need:

2 ounces of filtered water
1.5 cups of cubed pineapple
1 large orange, rind and seeds removed
¼ cup of fresh parsley
2 cups of spinach leaves

How to Make It:

Begin the prep for the juice by washing the parsley and the spinach leaves in a large colander. Leave colander in the sink, allowing the greens to dry while you prepare the other juice ingredients. If the pineapple is not cubed, cube it into pieces that will be a good fit for the juicer you use. Next, wash the orange, then peel the orange and remove any seeds. Break into sections. Add the pineapple, orange, parsley and spinach leaves to your juicer and juice the ingredients until the juice is ready. Mix the filtered water into the juice, making sure the juice and water are thoroughly combined. Fill a large glass with crush or cubed ice. Pour juice over ice and enjoy this pineapple orange flavored treat.

Recipe #29 – Sweet Cucumber Apple Green Juice Recipe

Spinach happens to be one of the healthiest vegetables out there, since it is filled with minerals, vitamins and anti-inflammatory properties. Some of the great vitamins and minerals your body will enjoy from spinach include vitamin E, zinc, calcium, vitamin C, vitamin A, folate, manganese, vitamin K and potassium. The addition of cucumbers and apples adds even more nutrition and the large amount of apples makes this green juice a wonderfully sweet concoction to sip on. You will fill as if you are having a nice treat as you enjoy this green juice.

What You'll Need:

2 large cucumbers, unpeeled
4 large handfuls of spinach leaves (you can substitute in Swiss chard too)
3 medium sized Fuji apples

How to Make It:

Start by washing the cucumbers thoroughly, leaving the peelings on them. Chop cucumbers into large pieces. Next, was spinach in a colander, making sure the spinach is well drained before you place it in the juicer. Wash the Fuji apples. Once washed, core the apples but do not remove the apple peels. Once fruits and veggies are prepared, add the cucumbers, spinach and Fuji apples to the juicer. After juicing has been completed, serve this juice immediately with a bit of ice to keep it cool. Enjoy the delicious sweetness.

Recipe #30 – Mint Pineapple Kale Green Juice Recipe

Kale is always a great ingredient to add to your green juices, since it is nutrient dense. It includes nutrients that help to build bones, detoxify the body, boost the immune system and support cardiovascular health. It can even help lower your risk for certain types of cancer. The addition of the pineapple is a wonderful, tasty treat. It adds plenty of flavor and also is good for you, improving digestion and reducing inflammation within your body. The added mint goes well with the pineapple and other ingredients in the green juice.

What You'll Need:

1 large Granny Smith apple
1 handful of mint leaves
½ lemon, rind removed
1 large cucumber
3 large leaves of kale
1 cup of chunked pineapple

How to Make It:

Place the mint leaves and the kale leaves into a colander, rinsing them carefully. Set aside and allow to dry. Take the Granny Smith apple and wash it for about 30 seconds. Remove the core from the apple but avoid removing skin. Cut apple into pieces. Cut a lemon in half, storing the unused half in the refrigerator. Peel the half you plan to use and ensure there are no seeds in the lemon. Wash the cucumber, leave it unpeeled, but cut it up into big chunks. In a juicer, place the Granny Smith apple, mint leaves, lemon, cucumber, kale leaves and the chunks of pineapple. Juice. Serve in a glass right away, enjoying the combination of delicious flavors.

Recipe # 31 – Body Restoring Green Juice Recipe with Coconut Water

If you have just been working out and you need a restorative drink, this green juice recipe is the perfect option. It helps to restore all the minerals, vitamins and electrolytes that you may lose while working out. It also works to help keep soreness and inflammation at bay. Every ingredient included offers great nutrition. The coconut water offers anti-bacterial and anti-aging benefits. The celery helps to lower blood pressure while the basil reduces the damage from free radicals and both the ginger and turmeric help to reduce inflammation. Some of the great nutrients included in this green juice include vitamin C, protein, vitamin K, phosphorus, copper, electrolytes, B complex vitamins, vitamin E, iron, potassium and calcium.

What You'll Need:

2 green apples, unpeeled
2 inches of turmeric
6 ribs of celery with leaves
4 large collard leaves
1 young coconut with white husk
1 knob of ginger
1 cup of basil leaves

How to Make It:

When choosing the coconut, ensure that the one you choose has a white husk, not a brown husk. Younger coconuts provide liquid that is richer in minerals. Crack the coconut open, straining out the coconut liquid. Set the coconut water to the side while working with other ingredients.

Wash basil and collard leaves in a colander and allow to drain and dry. Wash turmeric, celery, apples and ginger. Core apples, leave the peel in place, cutting the apples into big chunks. Cut the celery into chunks as well. Ginger should be cut into smaller pieces.

In a juicer, place the apples pieces, turmeric, celery chunks, collard leaves, ginger pieces and the basil leaves. Juice. Once juice is produced, place juice in a glass. Add in the coconut water that you set aside earlier. Mix well. Drink immediately.

Recipe #32 – Watermelon Ginger Cooling Green Juice Recipe

This green juice recipe is packed with nutritious goodness. The addition of watermelon adds nice flavor and watermelon also offers a variety of heart benefits. It is known to help reduce heart disease risk, protect against some cancers and is a powerful anti-inflammatory too. Lycopene is included in watermelon, which is an important antioxidant. With the combination of ingredients, some of the nutrients you will get from this juice include iron, manganese, magnesium, vitamin A, vitamin B6, molybdenum, vitamin K, folate and vitamin C.

What You'll Need:

1 large lemon, with the rind
1 large slice of watermelon, with the rind
1 bunch of parsley
1 inch of turmeric
1 inch piece of ginger
½ cucumber, with peel

How to Make It:

Wash parsley gently with cool water, allowing to drain

completely in a colander. Before slicing watermelon, wash rind carefully, since you will be using the rind. Was the lemon well too. Cut lemon into chunks and cube up the watermelon. Wash cucumber and then cut it in half. Place unused half in refrigerator to use later with another juice recipe. Cube remaining cucumber. Place the lemon with rind, watermelon with rind, parsley, turmeric, ginger and cucumber into the juicer, processing until juicing is complete. Enjoy at room temperature immediately.

Recipe #33 – Celery Watercress Green Juice Recipe

Watercress is often used as a garnish, but it has some great nutrients in it and is a great ingredient to add to your green juice recipes. It helps prevent migraines and may also help boost your immune system. The celery in the recipe helps the liver and lowers blood pressure, which apples aid with detoxification and help lower high cholesterol. Once all ingredients are combined, this green juice will provide you with vitamin K, vitamin A, vitamin E, magnesium, potassium, vitamin C, folic acid, copper and folate.

What You'll Need:

1 small lemon, rind removed
1 small lime, rind removed
1 bunch of watercress
1 medium head of celery
1 knob of ginger
3 medium sized Fuji apples

How to Make It:

Place the bunch of watercress in a colander, rinsing the leaves thoroughly and then allow them to drain. Peel the rind off the lemon and the lime, cutting them both into quarters. Wash celery and apples. Cut celery into medium sized chunks. Core the Fuji apples, cutting into pieces with the skin left on them. Ginger should be cut into smaller pieces as well. Once ingredients are prepared, add the lemon, lime, watercress, celery, ginger and apples to the juicer. Begin juicing. Place juice in a glass, enjoying the great flavors right away.

Recipe #34 – Cleansing Swiss Chard and Collard Leaf Green Juice Recipe

This green juice recipe is a wonderful one for cleansing the body. It helps to promote heart health by clearing arteries and helping to reduce cholesterol as well. The collard greens are great for cardiovascular support and they also help to prevent cancer. Swiss chard offers protection to the liver and even helps with the regeneration of pancreas cells. A wide variety of nutrients are included in this cleansing green juice, including zinc, folate, tryptophan, vitamin B6, vitamin C, beta carotene, vitamin E, choline, iron, vitamin K, calcium, potassium, protein and omega 3 fatty acids.

What You'll Need:

1 whole head of celery
2 inches of turmeric
½ beet
4 Swiss chard leaves
2 green apples
1 knob of ginger
1 piece of fennel
3 collard leaves
1 lime, rind removed

Combine the Swiss chard leaves and collard leaves in a colander, rinsing well. Wash the rest of the produce well. Once washed, begin chopping celery into cubes. Cut beat into quarters. Core the apples and then cut into cubes. Ginger should be cut into smaller pieces and lime should be cut in half. After preparing fruits and veggies, add the celery, turmeric, beet, Swiss chard leaves, green apple, ginger, fennel, collard leaves and lime to the juicer, processing completely. Pour juice into a cup and enjoy at room temperature as soon as possible.

Recipe #35 – Dandelion Green and Basil Green Juice Recipe

Dandelion greens can also be used to make a great green juice recipe. They pack plenty of nutrition in them, including potassium and calcium. Dandelion greens also work to help clean out the liver. All the other ingredients help give your body a boost as well. For example, the lime included helps give you a great dose of vitamin C while the basil helps to protect cell structures within the body. The turmeric helps to purify your blood and ginger improves overall circulation in the body. Enjoy great nutrients in this green juice, such as vitamin C, folate, iron, potassium, vitamin K, choline, beta carotene, protein and vitamin E.

What You'll Need:

1 inch of turmeric
2 green apples, unpeeled
3-4 leaves of Swiss chard
1 inch of ginger
1 lime, rind removed
½ bunch of dandelion greens
1 whole head of celery
1 cup of basil leaves

How to Make It:

Pull basil leaves off the stem, keeping leaves and disposing of stems. Then, place basil leaves, Swiss chard leaves and dandelion greens in a colander and rinse leaves well with cool water. Leave colander in sink so leaves drain completely. Wash turmeric and ginger, cutting both into small pieces. Apples should be washed, cored and cut into chunks. Remove the rind from the lime, cutting it in half. Wash the head of celery well, keeping the leaves. Cut celery up into cubes. Add the turmeric, apples, Swiss chard, ginger, lime, dandelion greens, celery and basil leaves to the juicer. Juice ingredients completely. Serve immediately, drinking this juice at room temperature.

Chapter 5: Your 7 Day Green Juicing Diet Meal Plan

Now that you have some excellent green juice recipes, you may be wondering how you can begin planning meals while you are on the green juice diet. What you should plan on is having a glass of green juice for each meal and it is nice to have a green juice snack while on the diet as well. Then, you can drink water and tea whenever you want. To get you started, the following is a helpful seven day green juicing diet meal plan that you can follow. After following it for a few days, you should find it easy to consider planning out your meals for each day as you continue on the diet.

Day 1:

Breakfast – Energizing Green Juice Recipe (Recipe #6)
Lunch – Kale and Cucumber Green Juice Recipe (Recipe #1)
Dinner – Beet and Cilantro Green Juice Recipe (Recipe #11)
Snack – Cabbage Broccoli Green Juice Recipe for Better Digestion (recipe #16)
Be sure to drink 8-10 glasses of water and tea if you

want it!

Day 2:

Breakfast – Spinach and Orange Green Juice Recipe
(Recipe #19)
Lunch – Sweet Mint Infused Green Juice Recipe (Recipe
#7)
Dinner – Broccoli Wheatgrass Green Juice Recipe (Recipe
#12)
Snack – Tropical Sweet Kale Green Juice Recipe (Recipe
#21)
Be sure to drink 8-10 glasses of water and tea if you
want it!

Day 3:

Breakfast – Pear Apple Papaya Green Juice Recipe
(Recipe #2)
Lunch – Carrot Cucumber Green Juice Recipe (Recipe #5)
Dinner – Celery Cucumber Spinach Green Juice Recipe
(Recipe #14)
Snack – Fill Me Up Green Juice Recipe (Recipe #8)
Be sure to drink 8-10 glasses of water and tea if you
want it!

Day 4:

Breakfast – Easy Apple Wheatgrass Green Juice Recipe (Recipe #18)

Lunch – Romaine Lime Green Juice Recipe (Recipe #9)

Dinner – Spinach and Kale Green Juice Recipe (Recipe #3)

Snack – Easy Cucumber Salad Green Juice Recipe (Recipe #13)

Be sure to drink 8-10 glasses of water and tea if you want it!

Day 5:

Breakfast – Watermelon and Cabbage Green Juice Recipe with Honey (Recipe #17)

Lunch – Vitamin Rich Green Juice Recipe (Recipe #10)

Dinner – Simple Green and Garlic Juice Recipe (Recipe #4)

Snack – Zucchini Cucumber Green Juice Recipe (Recipe #15)

Be sure to drink 8-10 glasses of water and tea if you want it!

Day 6:

Breakfast – Antioxidant Citrus and Spinach Green Juice

Recipe (Recipe #20)

Lunch – Delicious Watercress Green Bean and Spinach Green Juice Recipe (Recipe #25)

Dinner – Italian Style Green Juice Recipe (Recipe #23)

Snack – Strawberry and Tangerine Green Juice Recipe (Recipe #27)

Be sure to drink 8-10 glasses of water and tea if you want it!

Day 7:

Breakfast – Tangerine Broccoli Green Juice with Ginger Recipe (Recipe #26)

Lunch – Carrot and Kale Green Juice Recipe (Recipe #22)

Dinner – Bell Pepper Beet and Kale Green Juice Recipe (Recipe #24)

Snack – Sweet Cucumber Apple Green Juice Recipe (Recipe #29)

Be sure to drink 8-10 glasses of water and tea if you want it!

CPSIA information can be obtained
at www.ICGtesting.com
Printed in the USA
LVHW08s0526171018
593894LV00025B/234/P